EAT
TO
STAY
YOUNG

D1594202

EAT
TO
STAY
YOUNG

The Anti-Aging Program

Catherine Christie, Ph.D., R.D.
and Susan Mitchell, Ph.D., R.D.
with Debra Fulghum Bruce

KENSINGTON BOOKS
http://www.kensingtonbooks.com

KENSINGTON BOOKS are published by

Kensington Publishing Corp.
850 Third Avenue
New York, NY 10022

ISBN 1-57566-542-5

First Kensington Hardcover Printing: May, 1999
First Kensington Trade Paperback Printing: April, 2000
10 9 8 7 6 5 4 3 2 1

Printed in the United States of America

To my husband, Leo, whose steadfast encouragement, sense of fun, and love make my life a joy.

To my daughter, Tara Christie, my mother, Virginia Wilcox, my brother, Ben Wilcox, and my uncle, Ben Wilcox, for their unique perspectives that keep me grounded.

To my in-laws, Leo and Theresa Christie, and the Christie family, who provide a circle of family love and support.

And a special dedication to Joe and Rosemary Jacobs, without whom I would not be the person I am today.

Love to you all,
Catherine Christie, PhD, RD

To my husband, Charlie, whose sense of humor and joy for life keep me laughing and balanced.

To my in-laws, Dotty and Al Olsen, and the Olsen clan, who provide a circle of family love, values, and strong bonds.

To my brother, Dudley Mitchell, and my sister-in-law, Nancy Mitchell, who are pillars of love and support.

You are my greatest strength,
Susan Mitchell, PhD, RD

Acknowledgments

We are both fortunate to have a large circle of family, friends, and colleagues whose contributions make our writing and life in general fun and rewarding.

Many thanks to Debra Fulghum Bruce, whose creativity, enthusiasm, and consistent focus are incredible; Denise Marcil, our agent, for her dedication to our team and her unwavering support in all phases of this project; and Tracy Bernstein, our editor, and Laura Shatzkin, Director of Marketing and Promotion at Kensington, whose excitement over *Eat to Stay Young* was contagious and made our job as authors much easier.

For their belief in us, constant encouragement, love, and friendship, thanks to Sue and Buzz Crane; Jo Shuford Law, MS, LD, and Richard Law; Dan and Sylvia Schultz; Patty Thomas, RD, and Fred Fletcher; Carolyn and Bill Rayboun; Claire Lorbeer, MS, RD; Alice Rhatigan, MS, RD; Vilma Willard, MS, RD; Brenda Keen, RD; Toni Martin, MPH, RD; Lori Valencic, MS, RD; Juanita Bell; Eunshil Shim, MAg, RD; Jen Kring, RD; and Debra Waterhouse, MPH, RD. Thank you all for being who you are!

To Deanna Tompkins for reading the manuscript under tight deadlines; Heather McPherson for her help with the media; Kay and Virginia Braddock, whose e–mails mean so much; Marlene Stiwalt and Pam Smith, whose friendship and professionalism keep us running; Dorine Smith, RD, and Ellen Templeton Carroll, MS, RD, who never tire of listening and providing guidance; and Tandy Craig, Denise Davis, Suzy Wilson, Brenda Medlock Johnson, Deana Donoho, Martie Tucker, Jay Gaw, Laura Kittleson, Glenna and Dan Raidt, Linda Neuman, Novie Green, and Nancy Collins, MS, RD, who are the greatest cheerleaders anyone could ask for: thank you for touching our lives and hearts and for believing in us.

Contents

Introduction

Has this ever happened to you? Tiptoeing into your bathroom, you hope the well-lit mirror will not take notice so early in the morning. As you slowly turn your head, trying to avoid a face-off, something catches your eye. What? Jowls? A double chin? They were not there yesterday. A closer look into the eyes of the mirror reveals bubbly pouches of fat under your eyes and deeper creases on your forehead. It's coming. Your greatest fear—old age—is quickly making its approach.

Let's face it: While most people think of only two certainties in life—death and taxes—there is another certainty that is not frequently mentioned. In fact, you can defy it, deny it or denounce it, yet no matter how hard you try, you cannot avoid the inevitable truth—we are all getting older. While past generations more readily accepted the steady decline of physical and mental functioning many still associate with aging, studies reveal that most people today will continue to place a high value on being active and staying young.

We are nutrition and stress experts, and in all the work we do—leading seminars, counseling clients, and writing books—

we regularly interact with our clients and audiences to get a pulse on what people are seeking in their lives. Recently, while giving nationwide seminars, we conducted an extensive survey on aging in twenty major cities. The sample contained 1,000 participants between the ages of 25 and 75. More than two thirds of those who responded said they wanted to live to be 100, but only if they can stay healthy, be active, and look great. What did 90 percent of these participants say was stopping them from staying young? The number one obstacle identified was *stress.* It seems that we are so busy trying to do and be everything for everyone that we never have the time, or take the time, to nourish ourselves. Perhaps even more revealing, 93 percent of the participants said that daily stress ages them, specifically family, work, and financial stress.

We, too, have experienced the consequences of cumulative stress and how it makes you age:

Susan's Story

When Cathy and I wrote our first book, *I'd Kill for a Cookie,* I told how the unyielding stress of watching three members of my family—my mother, father, and brother—die within a period of three years had affected my eating and lifestyle habits. You see, I was one of those people whose appetite virtually shuts down when horrible events happen. During that terrible period in my life, I dwindled to 104 pounds because I felt too sick inside to eat. At five-six, you can imagine how I felt and looked—thin, gaunt, and old. I remember feeling numb and agonizing that though I had all these years of education and training, I could not stop the terminal diseases that took the lives of my loved ones. As I reflect on this stressful time, I definitely feel as if a part of me was lost with them, both emotionally and physically. I remember looking in the mirror, thinking, "I look and feel so much older than I really am.'' The dark, blackish-purple bags under my eyes were clear evidence of what lack of sleep or poor quality of sleep can do to a person. Signs of aging? I had it all: general fatigue, pasty skin, no sense of humor—stress-aging was happening right before my eyes.

Trust me, after much research and study, I know that it does not take a family catastrophe to stress-age. Today's harried world takes care of that quite nicely! Nonetheless, I also know that you hold the keys to looking and feeling young by recognizing these symptoms, identifying key stressors in your life, then making crucial changes to nourish yourself and regain control of your time and life. Our EAT Plan will guide you every step of the way—and it really works!

Cathy's Story

Work, work, work! No, I am not a workaholic, I just love what I do. Yet why is there always so much more to do than time to do it? Since Susan and I wrote *I'd Kill for a Cookie,* all of my work projects have expanded exponentially. It seems like just overnight our small seminar company went from three employees to eight, and the number of seminars each year has doubled. This resulted in twice the travel, half the time at home, and more preparation, reading, research, and updating. Add to this increased work load an abundance of radio interviews, print interviews, book signings, and more.

I'll admit that, yes, this is all part of being an author, but would someone tell me when the laundry will get done? Who will clean the house? And how will I ever find time to maintain the lawn? Perhaps, more important, when will there ever be time for me—to rest, exercise, read something for pleasure, or enjoy my family and friends? Add to this constant tension the stress of the VCR breaking down on the first day of a recent seminar and running to the store in between presentations to find a new one. While I'm away making this quick purchase, I call the office to find that two employees have resigned with only two weeks' notice, during which time I will be 1,000 miles away doing seminars. On top of these stressful interruptions, I make time on my one day at home for my yearly mammogram only to have the technician tell me, "Dr. Christie, I will need another picture because something looks funny in your left breast." Don't think it stops there! While obsessing on the statement "something looks funny in your left breast," I numbly travel to my next seminar site, get a wretched case of food poisoning, then spend from 11:00 P.M. until 4:00 A.M. throwing up. Keep reading! I get up at 5:30 A.M. to do a seminar on stress and eating . . . and that's just one week out of my life.

I did get a phone call later that week, informing me that my mammogram was normal, but take it from me, I know stress. I have seen stress-aging take its toll on my energy level, change the way I look and feel, and decrease my usual optimism and enthusiasm. Yet in the past few years the mirror has caught my eye, reminding me to slow down, take care of myself, and stop stress-aging before it gets out of hand—and the mirror does not lie! The good news is that stress-aging—that is, aging we can control—can be ended today . . . if you follow the easy steps in our EAT Plan.

Stay Young with the EAT Plan

Using our EAT Plan—your Energy-Action Team—we promise to show you breakthrough tools that will let you stay young no matter what your age or how you feel. Jumping off from the same scientifically based nutrition plan featured in our seminars, the EAT Plan is the first program ever written that uses food—something we all love anyway—to stay young and to stop stress-aging in its tracks. Imagine—eating to feel energetic, eating to sleep more soundly, eating to stay at a normal weight, eating to tame your hormones, eating to boost immunity, and even eating to look young again—our EAT Plan will help you do that and more.

The six steps in the EAT Plan—we call these Age Deactivators—build one upon the other to provide a cohesive, scientifically based nutritional blueprint to stop stress-aging. With each Age Deactivator, we will guide you through what to eat and when to eat it, as well as how to support your eating with the best herbs, supplements, exercise, and relaxation, using a myriad of charts, lists, and "smart steps" to help you incorporate the research into real life . . . yours. These Age Deactivators have helped thousands of seminar participants put the brakes on stress-aging and now they will help you.

The Six-Step EAT Plan Includes:

Age Deactivator 1: Eat Your Weedies: EAT to Stay Young and Disease-Free

Age Deactivator 2: Be Your Own Bodyguard: EAT to Improve Mental Attitude and Performance

Age Deactivator 3: Let Them Judge You by Your Cover: EAT to Look Young

Age Deactivator 4: Get Your Buns off the Back Burner: EAT to Stay Strong and Stand Tall

Age Deactivator 5: Find Relief for a Hard Day's Night: EAT to Sleep Well and Feel Rested

Age Deactivator 6: Gentlemen, Start Your Engines: EAT to Balance Hormones and Feel Young

The New Rules for Staying Young

We know the topic of aging is on everyone's mind. We also know that millions of men and women are sick and tired of feeling sick and tired and want to regain control of their youthful looks, energy, and effectiveness no matter what their age. In that regard, our six-step EAT Plan will be the new rules for staying young— no matter what your shape or condition.

The prescriptive advice in the EAT Plan may at first seem radical or inconsistent with some of the accepted principles of good health. We are Certified Nutrition Specialists, yet we do not believe in dieting, nor do we advocate the "no pain, no gain" theory of exercise and activity. We do believe in a specific real-life nutrition plan that nourishes you and can decrease stress and subsequently deactivate aging. Our prescriptive advice will replace the all-or-nothing mentality advocated by many popular health books today. And unlike many books based on mere specu-lation, the EAT Plan is based on the latest scientifically proven evidence.

By this time, you may be looking in a mirror, seeing how increasing years have changed your outer appearance. If you are wondering if your expanding waistline, sagging jowl, crow's-feet, laugh lines, thinning hair, gray hair . . . or no hair is partly a result of your daily battle with stress, you can count on it! *Even the slightest signs of aging are superactivated by daily stress,* which can rapidly wear down the body and weaken the immune system.

The fact is, the visible (crow's-feet and expanding waistlines) and not-so-visible (memory loss and chronic disease) signs of aging are much more controllable than you might think, and you will find solutions for these and other aging signs in this book.

The Secrets of Staying Young

Unlike books that paint a bleak picture of aging, we show you through compelling evidence the specific changes over which you have control—and yes, there are many. Think about the stressors that you are faced with daily—mortgage and utility payments, crowded freeways, traffic jams, declining mutual funds, increased taxes, upgrading, downsizing, child care, self care, elder care, health care . . . and who cares! Is it any wonder that most of us feel as if we need stronger defense mechanisms just to make it through the day?

Yet what happens when you add to your list of daily stressors a host of new physical changes—hair loss, weight gain, insomnia, menopause, high blood pressure, low bone density, high cholesterol, low sex drive, lumps, bumps, sags, bags . . . and gravity? Could some of these changes and decline in vitality be accentuated by unresolved or nagging stress? The answer is yes! We know from personal and professional experience: You may run, but you cannot hide. For all of us, stress will activate aging—if we don't start to nourish ourselves and gain control. Sure, you can usually coast to your mid-thirties with the luck of good genes. Yet there will come a guaranteed time of awakening—usually during midlife—when genetics subside and lifestyle factors take over. Surprisingly, research concludes that only about 30 percent of the characteristics of aging are genetically based; the remaining 70 percent are not.

I Don't Have to Look and Feel *Old?*

This is what we have in store for you: In Part I, we introduce you to cutting-edge information in the mind-body field of psychoneuroimmunology (PNI) and show how daily stress actually triggers the aging process to create unwanted changes. While the chemical changes brought on by stress can visibly influence how young you look and feel, stress is also a major factor in such serious health problems as memory loss, chronic headaches, depression, hypertension, obesity, allergies and asthma, heart disease, diabetes, and cancer.

How does stress activate aging, making you look and feel old before your time? For many of you, your day-to-day life may be very stressful, and this chronic stress can persist for weeks or even months. It is true that the immune system needs a certain amount of cortisol, which is the body's main stress-induced hormone. Yet when cortisol becomes elevated as with chronic stress and remains so for an extended period of time, it damages the cells that comprise your immune system.

Cortisol and the autonomic nervous system are both activated during stress. As a result of being bathed in the stress-related chemicals, the immune system is no longer capable of keeping infections, diseases, and free radicals at bay. The changes that result in the membranes of cells eventually lead to symptoms, disease, and accelerated aging.

Exposure to the invaders would have resulted in no problems, provided your immune system was strong. Yet as a result of chronic stress, your immune system simply will not work at full capacity. This breakdown in immune function literally activates internal and external changes associated with growing old.

With breakthrough research being done in the field of psychoneuroimmunology (mind-body interplay), no one can deny that stress negatively affects immune function whether we are young, old, or in between. In addition, stress produces such physical symptoms as muscle aches, headaches, back pain, tension, and digestive problems that make you *feel* old on a daily basis. Yet we can have control. Starting today, you can stop this unhealthy reaction called stress-aging, if you follow the six nutrition-based deactivators given in the EAT Plan.

Can an Apple a Day Keep the Doctor Away?

While studies show that we are more health conscious than ever, are we doing all we can to eat to stay young? In Part II of this book, you start our EAT Plan and learn what foods to eat and when to eat them. This plan is proven to help you stay young, increase vitality, and keep youthful good looks.

We give you surprising new research on specific vitamins that lower your chances of Alzheimer's disease as well as help the outer you by diminishing facial wrinkles and increasing collagen production. If you suffer from a racing mind and high anxiety and have difficulty sleeping, you will discover the specific foods that can calm you down and help you experience the healing sleep needed to produce human growth hormone that helps you stay young and feel alert. Likewise, our menu plan to help balance hormones can ease you through menopause without annoying symptoms, keep your bones strong, and even recharge your sexual vitality. Eating right, combined with exercise and other mind-body tools, will let you be on your way to deactivating stress-aging and feeling young again.

In our years of counseling clients and interacting in seminars, we have learned that each person is different with a unique set of needs. What works for one person may not help someone else. Therefore, we encourage you to use our flexible approach to derail stress-aging and stay youthful by choosing from the myriad of nutritional, psychological, spiritual, and physical options to find those that really work for you.

Happy Birthday!

Time triggers change, and change often happens gradually. What may have worked for you yesterday in looking and feeling young might not have the same effect now. Let today be your rebirth as you take time to reassess, refresh, and set new goals for your appearance, your health, and your overall productivity. It is time to love and nourish the person you are today—and the person you are to become.

Read on and let *Eat to Stay Young* with our extraordinary EAT Plan be your optimal guide to deactivate stress-aging and enjoy staying forever young!

Part I

. . .

Chapter 1

Escape the Daily Grind

"Take your mark . . . get set . . . go!" That's how Lorri describes a typical day—from the moment the alarm startles her at 5:30 A.M., until her youngest child is tucked in bed for the night, and she passes out with exhaustion—her life is an interminable race. The problem is that in the midst of running faster and harder each day to meet new clients, take care of her family's needs, or volunteer at school or in the community, this 40-year-old mother and free-lance journalist feels as if she never reaches the finish line.

"I think my nonstop life hit me the hardest when my eleven-year-old son, Ben, bought two gerbils. One gerbil stayed in the corner of the cage quietly eating his food, while the other gerbil ran constantly on the metal wheel connected to the cage. Ben couldn't stop laughing at the hyperactive gerbil, going around and around, getting nowhere. I was laughing, too, until my son said it reminded him of me."

There are times when most of us can identify with Lorri. We try to juggle all the responsibilities in life—kids, commitments, careers, and caregiving—but in the midst of our struggle to succeed or win in each area, we feel as if we are on a continuous treadmill stuck on high with no ''off'' button.

Think about it. Do you read a magazine while listening to the news, drinking a cup of coffee, and talking with your spouse or kids? This manner of behavior has become so common that it now has a name—time-stacking, which means ''juggling two or more activities at the same time''—and it has become a way of life for millions of men and women, especially those in relationships where both partners work. While juggling responsibilities, our personal time is virtually nonexistent, particularly with such intrusions as 24-hour e-mail, voice mail, faxes, and of course, the radio or television blaring in the background. Even when you take the phone off the hook and think you can finally have a respite, your office beeper or cellular phone alerts you to one more ''need'' you must answer.

In the midst of running this seemingly never-ending race we call ''life,'' you probably feel stretched to your limits. The good news is that you are not alone. According to the American Institute of Stress, 89 percent of the adults surveyed report having high levels of stress. In fact, at least 50 percent complained of this intense stress level at least once or twice a week, and more than 25 percent said they are stressed on a daily basis.

Lingo Lowdown

Simply stated, stress describes the many demands—physical, mental, emotional, or chemical—you experience each day. It includes the stressful situation (or stressor) and the symptoms you experience under stress (stress response). Stress can be negative (distress) or positive (eustress).

Study after study indicates that stress is skyrocketing, and you'd better fasten your seatbelt, because there is no indication that stress will level off anytime soon. In fact, many Americans report that they are *more* stressed now than 5 or 10 years ago. As David, a middle-aged attorney, said, "I get high anxiety just lying in bed thinking about what I have to do at the firm that day. Imagine how I feel at the end of my day!"

We don't have to imagine how David feels because we've heard it again and again from burnt-out clients and seminar participants. In fact, as clients have shared with us—job stress is the leading source of stress for adult Americans. Surveys validate this claim. In one, 78 percent of those questioned described their jobs as stressful, stating that their stress level has escalated over the past decade. In 1973, almost 40 percent of the workers surveyed said they were extremely satisfied with their jobs, fewer than 25 percent of all workers fall into this group today. If that isn't enough to turn your hair gray, consider this: Stress levels have also dramatically risen in other demographic groups including children, teenagers, and the elderly.

Comparing Apples to Pears

If you are wondering how daily stress affects you, take a look in the mirror. Better still, measure your waist. Has it had a "growth spurt" recently? If so, stress-aging may be taking its toll on you! In a paper published in the prestigious *New England Journal of Medicine,* Bruce McEwen, Ph.D., of Rockefeller University, identified eight physical indicators of an individual's personal stress load, such as blood pressure, cortisol levels, and abdominal fat. This "allostatic load" is the price our bodies pay for the ability to adapt to stress. Stressful life events, including daily wear and tear like traffic jams and family arguments, cause the body to release stress hormones such as cortisol. If these hormones are produced repeatedly or in excess because of chronic stress,

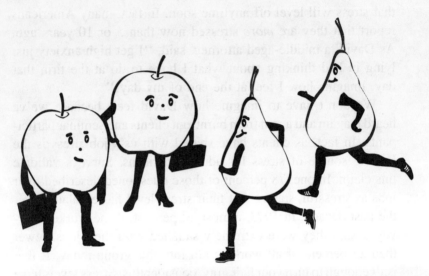

Figure 1.1

they create a gradual and steady cascade of harmful physiological changes to the body, including suppression of the immune system (which means we catch colds and flu much more easily), and increased insulin levels, which are tied to greater fat deposits around the abdomen. These fat deposits give an apple shape to our body, and this shape has been tied to a greater risk for heart disease, diabetes, high blood pressure, and certain forms of cancer. Even the brain can be affected. In fact, McEwen concluded that a lifelong allostatic load may accelerate changes in the brain that can lead to memory loss.

For right now, just keep McEwen's stress study tucked away in your memory bank. We will show you some surefire ways to stop these physical and mental effects of stress-aging in our EAT Plan, outlined later in the book. But keep reading, and let's focus on the impact time-stacking and increasing stress have on your life.

Think about where you go for lunch each day. Wait a minute . . . you say you don't eat lunch? Again, you aren't alone. Surveys show that most of us are so pushed and stressed that we do not take time to stop and enjoy this midday meal anymore. According to a revealing poll from the National Restaurant Association, 40 percent of all workers surveyed do not take a break away from the office for lunch. Other surveys have shown that the lunch hour isn't even close to an hour but more like 29 to 36 minutes. Many of us just skip lunch completely since we are so squeezed for time between our work and home life. It has become customary to use this short break in the day to run errands, have a haircut or dental appointment, or catch up with paperwork at our desk.

So, if we don't take time for lunch, what are the current eating trends? Studies conducted by the NPD Group, a consumer research organization that tracks how America eats, confirm that lunch, not breakfast, is the one meal we usually skip. (Wouldn't that make Mom proud after years of reminding us to eat breakfast!) Of those who do each lunch, the NPD Group reported that many are brown-bagging it; 43 percent of men and 34 percent of women bring a sack lunch from home at least once every two weeks. Why? Well, perhaps Janis, a successful investment banker who thrives on a homemade PBJ each day, has the answer: "It's easier, less expensive, and you can eat at your desk while reviewing your afternoon appointments."

Yes, it may seem easier and less expensive, but what cumulative effect does constant juggling, time-stacking, and the resulting stress have on us? You know the answer—it makes us look and feel old . . . years before our time. Or to put it more succinctly, running faster and harder on this nonstop treadmill we call life causes us to stress-age.

So, Who's the Fairest of Us All?

As much as you might try, you cannot hide stress-aging, and a quick look in the bathroom mirror says it all. Listen to what some of our seminar participants have said upon identifying that intimate link between daily stress and the outward signs of aging:

"After not sleeping for two weeks during a company audit, I awoke one day and felt like I had aged ten years with saggy skin and swollen pouches under my eyes."

"When my wife and I separated last year, my hair seemed to turn gray and thin overnight."

"My fifteen-year-old son has hormone havoc, and I have the resulting love handles from eating to soothe my frayed nerves."

"Between balancing my job teaching school with raising kids and caring for my aging parents, I never have time to care for myself, and I have an abundance of cellulite to prove it."

"While some people may have laugh lines, I have worry wrinkles—deep crevices around my eyes and mouth that I know came from years of anxiety, worrying about my marketing business."

Perhaps this one is the most revealing of stress-aging:

"When my husband and I went to our twenty-year high school reunion, a man walked over and said I looked familiar. Then he asked if I had taught him English in tenth grade. I was humiliated! It was a guy I had dated a few times in high school, and he didn't recognize me. Sure, I had a successful chain of restaurants in three cities, but I looked hard and haggard. I felt old."

As we share in our seminars, dark undereye circles, pasty skin, thinning or gray hair, love handles, cellulite, and not-so-funny laugh lines are definitely distressing. Yet there is a far more serious consequence of stress-aging: Stress impairs our resistance to such invaders as cold germs, high cholesterol, or even cancer cells.

Science now recognizes that the mind and body are interconnected to an extent far surpassing previous assumptions and that physical health and emotional well-being are closely linked. In simpler terms, daily stress leads to emotional turmoil that can shock an immune system into a downward spiral, resulting in chronic or serious illness. Is it any wonder that after living in our fast-paced, time-stacking society, a startling 75 to 90 percent of all the doctor visits made annually are for stress-related problems?

Just the Facts

Stress has been linked to the following illnesses:

Allergies, asthma, and hay fever	High blood pressure
Arthritis	Migraine headaches
Back pain	Temporomandibular joint syndrome (TMJ)
Cancer	Tension headaches
Chronic pain	Stroke
Heart disease	Ulcers

The EAT Plan Is Your Fountain of Youth

Today, thanks to scientific and medical research, we have a better idea of how stress affects every aspect of our lives. While there is no quick fix for years of ignoring your immune system, our EAT Plan will help bring a dramatic difference in the way you look and feel. We aren't just talking about optimal health but also about improving memory and learning, increasing energy, promoting sounder sleep and better sex, and gaining control over your appetite—and that's just the beginning!

"Okay. I see that stress has plumped me up, zapped my energy, and makes me forget my name, and that's on a good day! But why do some people look so old before their time, while their friends are still carded for beer at local convenience stores?'' That's a good question, and one that scientists still have not figured out completely. For the past few decades, researchers have been intrigued with this very question, looking at why we age and hoping to find that magic cure. The fact is, the outlook for extending lifespan is remarkably better than in the past.

With varying interpretations of how the aging process is triggered, scientists do agree on one point: Aging is a complex process that is controlled by both environmental factors and genetics. Age researchers contend that various stress situations may to some extent actually control how fast we age. In our seminars, we prefer to say that aging can be ''activated'' or ''deactivated'' by different factors, which we will explain fully throughout this book.

Ginny attended one of our seminars last year. For years, this mother of three teenage daughters was often mistaken for being ''one of the girls'' instead of Mom. Yet in the past year Ginny had undergone surgery twice for precancerous conditions, had developed hypertension (high blood pressure), and was showing early signs of thinning sun-damaged skin. She was definitely looking for some magic cure to help her regain control of what was happening to her looks and her health.

As we shared with Ginny and the rest of the seminar participants, there are several theories on aging. One theory suggests that cell loss is a major determinant of the aging process. Cells have been found to have finite lives. Most are replaced through cell division but at a decreasing rate over time and a maximum of about 100 divisions. Brain cells (neurons) and heart cells (myocytes) do not divide at all, and when these are lost, well, they are gone forever. Interestingly, as cell numbers decline so do their end products such as collagen and elastin, which provide resilience for your bones, muscles, and skin.

These wear-and-tear theorists believe that merely living will age us, because of the nature of our normal metabolism. When the body takes in oxygen and nutrients and converts these to energy, it produces harmful by-products called free radicals, which race around oxidizing other molecules in the body and changing their structure. Not only are free radicals produced, but over time your body's hormone and enzyme levels decline.

Just like your love-crazed teenager in spring, free radicals are highly unstable and eager to pair with the next available molecule. But when they meet, the union sets off a negative stream of events. For example, through this oxidation process, LDL cholesterol (the bad kind that resembles solid yellow shortening in a can) is produced and gets deposited as plaque right smack on your artery walls.

The negative effects of these free radicals also include high blood pressure, high cholesterol, and increased glucose levels, not to mention aging skin, wrinkles, and a host of others. Although genetics are the key players in aging, certain environmental factors, such as tobacco smoke and ultraviolet light, which stimulate the production of more free radicals, can influence how quickly this occurs.

Anatomy 101

Let's say you just bought the car of your dreams and decide to drive it to the beach, where you have rented a house for the summer. When you get there, you find out there is no garage, so your new car is going to be exposed to the hot sun, wind, and blowing sand. If your car is exposed to these elements over time, what happens to it? You got it. It starts to rust. Think of free radicals as your body's "rust," after it is exposed to sunlight, pollution, smoke, and other elements.

Eat Less to Stay Young?

At a time when eating disorders are epidemic, we almost hate to share this aging theory and give some people a "reason" not to eat. Still, research has shown that modestly restricting the calorie intakes of monkeys and rats produces a more efficient metabolic rate. While the restriction of calories may result in a lower body temperature and subsequent decrease in oxygen consumption, not all of the questions have been answered. Perhaps the more efficient metabolism may mean fewer free radicals and thus a longer life, but honestly, while controlling calories makes sense, this theory is still speculative.

If what current research suggests is true, perhaps an antiaging hormone or drug could someday have the same effect as caloric restriction. At this time, fascinating studies are being conducted to see if low dosages of hormones or high dosages of vitamins can reduce the effects of free radicals. An excellent example is the comprehensive work being done by the National Institute of Aging on melatonin, which can affect sleep cycles; DHEA (dehydroepiandrosterone), a product of the adrenal glands that converts to estrogen and testosterone; and HGH (human growth hormone), which affects bone and organ development as well as metabolic rate.

"An antiaging pill? When? Where? How much?" Whoa! Slow down here. Before you run to the local pharmacy in search of a new "youth" pill, remember that many factors may activate aging. Now put your keys down and keep reading because on the opposing side of this research are a myriad of scientists who hold strongly to the theory that aging must still be linked with our genes.

Are Your Genes Worn Out Yet?

Only you know how your genes fit! How did your mother or grandmother age? Take a look at them or their pictures. To be quite honest, what you see is probably what you are going to look like. Is that a scary thought? What about Dad, his brothers, or his father? Genetics do seem to play a significant role in how we age, and gene theorists state that cell division holds the key to the mystery of aging. When the process is disrupted, immune problems set in. Some researchers theorize that cells have a clock-like lifespan and will divide until the clock winds down. An even newer theory suggests that a stress-response gene plays a role in aging as it regulates the body's repair and maintenance.

At the tip of every chromosome (a bundle of DNA where genetic information is stored in a cell), is a "telomere" that gets a little bit shorter every time the cell divides. Scientists theorize that telomeres thus help regulate how many times a cell divides before it dies. When the telomere eventually becomes too short to protect the chromosome, the cell can no longer divide, and it dies. In this light, the telomere seems to act as a biological clock that stops cell division and activates aging.

In landmark studies at the University of Texas Southwestern Medical Center, researchers have zeroed in on the role of telomerase, the enzyme that regulate telomeres. Amazingly, when they added telomerase to the chromosomes of cells, the cells continued to divide and showed no signs of aging or dying. Their work could possibly lead to breakthrough drugs that will stop cells from dying and preserve the functioning of body parts that normally breakdown as we age. By keeping the cells alive and dividing, it may be possible to control age-related disorders ranging from skin wrinkling to some types of blindness and perhaps even heart disease and autoimmune diseases like lupus or multiple sclerosis (MS).

Immunity's Role in Aging

Not only is aging a hot topic for scientific research and debate, but so is immunity, particularly the ways in which a strong immune system can help keep you healthy and looking young. You don't have to travel farther than your television set to hear about the latest health study linking stress to a depressed immune system or the degenerative and chronic diseases associated with stress and aging.

As you will learn in this book, your immune system craves attention—the healthy attention that can come when you start our EAT Plan. But first let's look at how the immune system can help you to stay young—or age you quickly. The immune system is your body's own healing system and also the body's natural defense against infection and disease. Its main function is to distinguish itself (you) from nonself (a host of invaders) through a complex network of antibodies, proteins, and specialized cells. Your spleen and thymus are crucial organs of the immune system and produce white blood cells called lymphocytes. Other white blood cells include natural killer (NK) cells and macrophages. All of these cells have a mission, which is to keep you healthy at all costs by attacking and destroying foreign materials.

Anatomy 101

Lymphocytes act like your personal bodyguards, traveling throughout the body keeping an eye open for any foreign invader. Corresponding troops in the lymph nodes and spleen stay on red alert—ready to go to war at a moment's notice.

Invaders take the form of bacteria, viruses, parasites, and fungi, all of which are called antigens. When the immune system fails to function as it should, and mistakenly attacks your own body, the result is the development of autoimmune diseases such as arthritis, allergy, asthma, lupus, or multiple sclerosis. If your immune system is depleted, your body is at risk of being over-whelmed by invading bacteria and viruses, resulting in cancer or other life-threatening diseases.

Changes in levels of hormones produced by daily stress can negatively affect immune function, particularly the nerve cells connecting the brain to other vital organs. The nerve cells are directly involved in making immune system cells, and when stress levels increase, it results in an overproduction of stress hormones that tear down or weaken our immune system. The result? We stress-age.

Not only is stress an important factor for the development of disease in and of itself, but it also affects your health and aging by influencing the lifestyle choices you make, such as whether you smoke or drink, the foods you eat or don't eat, your bedtime, exercise patterns, and a host of other habits. Deleterious habits not only increase your risk for diseases such as cancer but also activate stress-aging. Alarmingly, the sum of poor lifestyle habits is more harmful to your body than one habit by itself.

It's Time for Innercise

"Innercise? Don't you mean exercise?" That was Sandy's response when we told her that to stay young, she needed to get in touch with her inner beliefs and emotions and take time for personal or inner renewal. Sandy, a competitive real estate broker and weekend warrior, had been doing step aerobics daily for years. Not only did she work out, she also watched what she ate, choosing an array of fruits, vegetables, and low-fat foods that would make any nutritionist proud. Nonetheless, Sandy had some inner turmoil that was causing her great stress, and it was taking its toll on her immune system. Divorced for more than two years, Sandy still held a lot of hostility and anger inside and would lash out at someone when they least expected it. She could not figure out why she had been sick with colds and viruses in the past few months and just could not seem to shake them.

Our goal was to convince Sandy to think about the relationship between her inner attitude and daily thoughts and the effect these have on her body and mind. This mind-body interaction is called psychoneuroimmunology (PNI), and a tremendous amount of research is being conducted in this field to determine the links between stress, aging, emotions, and disease.

Lingo Lowdown

Psychoneuroimmunology means mind-body interplay. *Psycho-* stands for "mind," *neuro-* for the "neuroendocrine system" (the nervous and hormonal systems), and *immunology* for the "immune system."

Those on the cutting edge of psychoneuroimmunology contend that many influences are at work in each of us either to keep us well or allow us to get sick. Scientific evidence suggests that factors such as stress, negative feelings, and lack of social support can influence both immune status and function, as well as lead to stress-aging and disease onset and progression. Although still preliminary, research also suggests a role for psychological factors in autoimmune diseases such as allergies, arthritis, and multiple sclerosis.

Robert Ader, Ph.D., a research psychologist at the University of Rochester School of Medicine, is considered the founder of PNI. In the late 1970s, Ader performed some of the first studies on the link between the immune system and the central nervous system. Herbert Benson, M.D., another great pioneer of PNI, is the author of *Timeless Healing* (Scribner, 1996) and president of the Mind/Body Medical Institute at the Harvard-affiliated Beth Israel Deaconess Medical Center. He has suggested that the practice of medicine is like a three-legged stool, where the legs of surgery and medications are balanced by spiritual self-care. Thanks to the work of Ader, Benson, and a host of other brilliant researchers, many studies are now focused on the mechanisms by which the mind and emotions affect physical well-being. For someone who has difficulty getting pregnant, can't shake a lingering cold, or is concerned about an increased risk for heart disease, cancer, or diabetes, these lifesaving studies can outline how emotional distress may be a crucial barrier to wellness.

The Pitfalls and Pratfalls of Stress

"I've heard enough, thanks!" Kim could not wait until the first part of our seminar was over. This 34-year-old mother of twin boys had already closed her notebook, tuned us out, and was ready to exit through the side door during the break. "If it's not the twins, then it's my job. If not my job, then it's the school or neighbors or in-laws. I'm always uptight, anxious, and stressed about something. From the sound of these aging theories, I might as well go home and write my obituary."

We talked Kim into waiting another hour, and by the time we explained our EAT Plan and how it could stop her stress-aging today, she was convinced that this was the ticket to feeling young again. One revealing study we shared with Kim and the other attendees was conducted at the Behavioral Medicine Research Center in Durham, North Carolina, which evaluated whether "role overload" could affect our minds or bodies. Researchers found that working women with children at home, independent of marital status or social support, excrete greater amounts of the stress hormone cortisol and experience higher levels of home strain than those without children at home. Kim later told us that as a working mother of energetic eight-year-old boys, she did not need a scientific study to predict this outcome!

Yet another study hit home for Kim, a computer salesperson for a tri-county area. The *Lancet* reported that long commutes and extended work hours may overactivate the sympathetic nervous system, which kicks in the fight-or-flight response. Now, the fight-or-flight response is great if you are fighting wild animals, but in our daily lives such symptoms as an increased heart rate and increased production of stress hormones will only serve to make us old—fast.

Lingo Lowdown
The fight-or-flight response is a physical response controlled by our hormones and nervous system that prepares us to fight or flee our stressor.

Not only do you have to get in control of kids, career, chaos, and commitment in your lives, but there is another risk factor for stress-aging that you may be unaware of—the type D personality. Researcher Johan Denollet, Ph.D., of the University of Antwerp in Belgium, has labeled people who are negative, insecure, and distressed as "type D" personalities. Denollet suggests that these people are three times more likely to suffer a second heart attack than "non-D types."

Still other findings reveal that long-term caregiving may set you up for decreased immunity and increased chance of disease. A study done on caregivers of Alzheimer's patients found these people had a poor immune response as measured by the number of killer cells. This decease in immunity lasted even three years past the end of their caregiving.

Perhaps the most revealing research on stress is being done with breast cancer patients. Ohio State University researchers have concluded that the stress women experience after breast cancer diagnosis and surgery can weaken their immune response. According to a report in the *Journal of the National Cancer Institute,* this study continues to document the link between conditions of high stress and low immunity. Barbara Andersen, professor of psychology and researcher at Ohio State's Comprehensive Cancer Center and Institute of Behavioral Medicine Research, and her colleagues studied women who underwent breast cancer surgery. Before the women began follow-up therapy, they completed an extensive questionnaire intended to gauge their stress levels and were then ranked either high- or low-stress. Blood was drawn from women in both groups and tested for different indicators of immune status. The results were astounding: Women in the high-stress group had 15.4 percent fewer NK cells (vital killer cells that help fight disease) than those in the low-stress group.

Don't Worry, Be Happy

As we shared in the introduction, according to Dr. John Rowe, director of the MacArthur Foundation Consortium on Successful Aging, about 30 percent of aging is genetically based. That means the other 70 percent is not! Perhaps it is this 70 percent of aging that can be intimately linked to stress and lifestyle habits—habits that we have the power to *change.*

"Why didn't someone tell me about this stress-aging theory ten years ago before I had children?" Jennifer, a dental hygienist and mother of two, was also taking care of her 80-year-old father who had diabetes. She felt as if we were talking about her life in each study that was discussed. Take heart, Jennifer. Raising kids, caregiving, and a stressful career are not going away anytime soon, but we are going to teach you easy ways to take control of life's stressors with our EAT Plan. First we need to remind you that mental and physical activities such as innercise (checking out inner emotions) and exercise (climbing those stairs at work and taking long brisk walks with your children after school) will work together to boost brain function and keep you young. Education is important, too, so continue to learn all you can to keep those brain cells charged. According to Marilyn Albert, Ph.D., of Harvard Medical School, high levels of stress hormones may harm brain cells and cause atrophy in an area important to memory known as the hippocampus.

Throughout this book we will be talking more about your immune system, tagging certain negative lifestyle factors as Immune Busters, as well as discussing what you can do for healing using our list of Immune Boosters. But before we continue, let's consider your status right now. Is your immune system under attack from your hectic and harried lifestyle, or are you in control? Use the following checklist to find out:

Immune Busters

Check each of the following Immune Busters that may be negatively affecting your natural immunity. Give yourself 1 point if this describes you, and 0 if it does not. Add up your score to see where you stand.

_____ 1. too little sleep
_____ 2. negative attitude
_____ 3. depression
_____ 4. repressed feelings
_____ 5. sense of worthlessness
_____ 6. poor diet
_____ 7. extreme exercise
_____ 8. very little exercise
_____ 9. loneliness
_____ 10. recent job loss or lack of employment
_____ 11. job dissatisfaction

_____ 12. shift work
_____ 13. recent death of a loved one
_____ 14. caregiving to a chronically ill person
_____ 15. marital separation and/or divorce
_____ 16. exposure to environmental pollutants
_____ 17. overexposure to sunlight
_____ 18. smoker
_____ 19. heavy alcohol use
_____ 20. long-term medication usage

Now total up your score:

14–20: Immunity busted! Call in the tag team. Your score indicates a threatened immunity. Read on to learn about specific age-deactivators, including smart foods that can help lessen the threat of attack on your immune system.

7–13: Your score is on the edge and you may be getting run down. Check out the EAT Plan to find easy ways to strengthen your immune system.

1–6: Immunity boosted! Today your immunity is not under siege. To keep your immune system boosted, follow the EAT Plan and continue to enjoy staying young.

You Are Not Alone!

If you scored Immunity Busted, you are not alone. Millions of men and women are suffering from a lifetime of chronic stress and negative lifestyle choices. Now don't think that we'd give you all of these revealing studies on stress-aging without telling you some good news—and there is some exciting news! No matter how out of balance your life is, much of the breakdown of the immune system can be stopped and even healed. As you will learn in the EAT Plan—you can deactivate aging now with food and supplement choices, as well as a healthy combination of regular exercise, innercise, and an optimistic outlook on life.

As you will learn in Chapter 2, optimism has a profound influence on immunity. Take laughter, for example. Scientists have found that laughing—something most of us do every day—can produce a state of positive stress, or what is called eustress. While studying laughter's effect on the immune system, researchers at Loma Linda University in California showed a video of a comedian. Blood samples drawn during and after the video both showed significant increases in various measures of immune function, particularly T-cells and NK (natural killer) cells, and a lowered level of the stress hormone cortisol, which suppresses the immune system. The researchers concluded that laughter creates its own physiological state with positive changes in the immune system.

Lingo Lowdown

Eustress Is Positive Stress

Having a party	A pay raise	Getting engaged
Graduating from college	Going on a cruise	Winning a contest
Finding out you are expecting a baby	Getting a promotion	Buying a new home

---

Beyond optimism and laughter, positive physiological and psychological benefits have even been linked to the presence of Fido and Fluffy in your home. Researchers suggest that decreases in blood pressure, heart rates, and stress levels, as well as increases in emotional well-being and social interaction are among the healthful benefits of the human-animal bond.

The EAT Plan Is Your Fountain of Youth

Now that you have a basic understanding of why you look and feel the way you do from those in the know—researchers and scientists studying the link between stress and aging—go ahead and turn the page.

Take the leap to Chapter 2 to discover how "soul food" is one type of nutrition you must have to keep immune balance and stay forever young.

Chapter 2

Make Time for Soul Food

Jody, a successful tax attorney, caught up with us after a seminar last year for assistance in coping with the stress in her life. This well-educated woman had just turned 40 and was at least that many pounds over a healthy weight for her height and build.

We talked for a minute about her medical history, and then asked about her career, family, diet, lifestyle, and activities. Her story was one that as nutritionists we hear daily: too much work, not enough personal time, too many grab-it-and-go meals and low nutrient snacks, not enough exercise, too much stress, no time for fun or friends, not enough meaningful experiences, and so on.

But Jody also said something that we all need to take seriously as she unhappily acknowledged, "In trying so hard to make a living, I've neglected to make a life."

Aren't we all like that? We get so caught up in the pressures of our goal-oriented society that the only measurement we have of personal fulfillment lies in wealth and status. In our free time—what little there is—we spend millions of dollars on fitness equipment, diet foods, antiaging creams, and the latest fad supplements, trying to look and feel young again. There must be a better way!

If you're feeling old before your time, you are probably well aware of the anguish it can cause. Perhaps you have blamed your lack of energy or enthusiasm on the frantic pace of life. But if we are emotionally drained, life's stressors, when they hit, are greatly magnified. Most of us have experienced fatigue, weariness, and ultimately, burnout. We want relief, results, and healing but do not know where to turn, and it often seems next to impossible to rejuvenate our spirit after doing daily battle in today's world.

Lingo Lowdown
Burnout: A state of physical and emotional exhaustion.

Discovering Soul Food

Take it from us—life does not have to be so exhausting! In the EAT Plan, explained on pages 97–253, we will speak frequently of the need for "soul food" as a way to settle your inner spirit and deactivate aging, and we are not referring to the traditional Southern cuisine of fried chicken, turnip greens, and cornbread—as delicious as that may sound. Rather, we are talking about the fulfillment needed to satisfy our inner hunger.

"I didn't realize that this was a religious plan. That's not going to work for me." Jake was a seminar participant who wanted immediate help in stopping stress-aging. In the past year, this 39-year-old father of four had invested his life savings into a car leasing business, then just found out that his wife was pregnant again—with twins. Don't worry! While many of us equate the word "spirituality" with religion and use words such as faith, hope, and love to describe it, spirituality does not have to be associated with a religious faith. In fact, you can nourish your inner spirit without having to believe in a religious doctrine.

Let's just say that for the purposes of this book, spirituality is an inner intangible force that allows you to cope with life's challenges. This force can stem from a belief in one's god or other external guiding force or perhaps from resources within, and that is where the term "soul food" comes in.

Psychotherapist James Hillman was one of the first to rediscover the soul as an important concept in psychotherapy, but it was theologian and author Thomas Moore, one of Hillman's followers, who identified "soul-sickness" as an epidemic sweeping our planet. "Emptiness; meaninglessness; vague depression; disillusionment about marriage, family, relationships; a loss of values; yearning for personal fulfillment; a hunger for spirituality" are all symptoms Moore identifies when people "lose the soul."

In *Care of the Soul* (HarperCollins, 1992), Moore maintains that the soul has to do with genuineness and depth, as when we say certain music has soul or a remarkable person is soulful. Soulfulness is linked to life in all its particulars—good food, satisfying conversations, genuine friends, and meaningful experiences that stay in the memory and touch the heart.

We strongly believe that when you care for your soul and nurture your inner spirit, other areas of life, including gaining control over stress-aging, can be more easily changed. And this care of the soul means giving meticulous attention to our daily actions—what we think, what we feel, what we eat, and yes, even our friends, career choice, and what we do in our downtime.

Getting Body and Soul in Sync

How does soul-sickness relate to looking and feeling young? As we will share in the EAT Plan, when you can admit to needing inner fulfillment, take stock of what is missing from life, and then get in touch with "matters of the heart"—faith, hope, intimacy, passion, belief, responsibility, relationships, and optimism—you can begin to manage your life and deactivate stress-aging. Today, thanks to new scientific research, we have a better understanding of spirituality and its effect on human beings. Researchers have looked at the benefit of these "matters of the heart" and found that people who practice them tend to live longer and stronger than those without them. In a number of scientific studies, researchers found that practicing such ideals in daily life was tied to heightened immunity, the ability to deal with life's stressors, and increased health and longevity.

Great men are they who see that spiritual is stronger than any material force, that thoughts rule the world.
—Ralph Waldo Emerson

You may know personally that when your spiritual side is ignored, you experience a gnawing emptiness such as Moore describes that you desperately try to fill with destructive life-style habits—cigarette smoking, overeating, too much alcohol, no time for family or friends, or late nights with poor sleep. Too often the results are lack of energy, health problems, and an overall feeling of malaise. When the pieces of life's puzzle are all in place, as you will learn with each of our Age Deactivators, you will experience a vital balance between your body, mind, and spirit.

From Stone Age to New Age

Perhaps you are thinking that the mind-body interplay we speak of is some "New Age" concept. Actually, the belief that one's mind and spirit can have a dramatic effect on the physical body is not a new revelation at all. In the 2,000-year-old Hippocratic writings, there are observations that there is a measure of conscious thought throughout the body. And today, Dr. Dean Ornish's successful program for reversing heart disease is based on a disciplined and meditative lifestyle that focuses on inner peace along with exercise and a healthful nutrition plan. Bill Moyers also confirmed the spiritual dimension of health in his ground-breaking PBS-TV series and book *Healing and the Mind.* Moyers reported that there is, in fact, a relationship between our emotions or spiritual state and our bodies and tells how, in China, the physician is thought of as a gardener. The physician teaches the patient to be a gardener and helps the patient understand how to summon the healing faculties of her body for recovery.

Stop Singing the Blues

"Well, if my thoughts and personality are related to my health, then I better review my will," Mark told us at a recent seminar. "I've always been a negative person. It's a genetic trait because I come from a long line of pessimists." This 32-year-old banker rarely cracked a smile during our day-long seminar and refused to join his colleagues in the personality assessment questionnaire. He even emphatically turned thumbs down on our suggestion that he needed to do some soul searching before he could start the EAT Plan, saying, "I've tried stuff like that before and it never works for me."

It's interesting how some people can have a glass that is half full, while others complain that their glass is always half empty. We all know people who always make "lemonade out of lemons," and "bless their mess," while others are perpetually sucking on a lemon, ready to pounce on any negative intrusion in their lives.

Yet maybe Mark is partially right. Perhaps he can blame his

depressed genes for his sourpuss outlook and half-empty glass. For years, researchers have tried to determine the relationship between genetics and environment in answering the questions: Is there an optimism gene which predetermines your personality and outlook on life? Do early childhood experiences drive your view of life? Or can you change your outlook on life when you're an adult? Surprisingly, the answers are yes, yes, and yes!

A revealing study of 854 female twin pairs was conducted in 1997 by Kenneth Kendler, M.D., from the Virginia Institute for Psychiatric and Behavioral Genetics and reported in the *American Journal of Psychiatry*.

Researchers identified six categories of social support which they measured:

1. Family problems—relationship difficulties such as making too many demands, being critical, or creating tension.
2. Family support—caring, encouragement, and assistance.
3. The presence and number of confidants a person has to rely on.
4. Social integration—the frequency of contact and attendance at clubs and organizations.
5. Friend problems—relationship difficulties such as making too many demands, being critical, or creating tension.
6. Friend support—number of friends, level of caring, and assistance.

The levels of these six factors did not change much over time (a five-year interval was studied). Both genetic and environmental factors accounted for twin resemblance in family or relative problems and family or relative support. Interestingly, the number of confidants and social integration had the strongest genetic influences. The authors concluded that genetics or inborn personality traits powerfully influence the way we create social relationships throughout life. David Lykken, a professor of psychology at the University of Minnesota in Minneapolis, also studied twins and found similar results. Even twins who were raised in vastly different environments had pretty much the same levels of well-being as those who were brought up together.

The Pollyanna Paradigm

What does this mean for people like Mark, who blame their family tree for a negative outlook on life? Genetics may indeed play a significant part in how you view life. Based on recent scientific tests, we know that our capacity for happiness is somewhat genetically preset, and happiness has less to do with events that occur, both good and bad, than with how we perceive those events. Nonetheless, the good news is that researchers also agree that we can reset our happiness set point with therapy or even with everyday activities that bring pleasure such as reading a book, gardening, working on a hobby, enjoying a cup of tea, or eating a favorite food.

While this may sound too easy to work, you may want to practice smiling if you are typically a toxic or critical person. Study after study continues to show that negative emotions such as chronic anger, pessimism, mistrust, cynicism, and depression throw the immune system into such a battered state that it is difficult to resist disease. Smiling is the body's signal that you are happy, optimistic, and in a positive emotional state. If you "fake it until you make it," negative emotions can be turned into a more positive view. Scientists have also found that negative people are more prone to develop certain diseases, and recover more slowly, than their positive counterparts.

> **Just the Facts**
> Norman Cousins was the first to promote laughter as an anti-dote to disease. While editor of the *Saturday Review,* Cousins was diagnosed with a serious connective tissue disease. Although his doctors said that it was incurable, he was determined to get well. During his journey to find a cure for his ailment, Cousins discovered that laughter actually affected his body chemistry in a positive, healing way. He filled his life with movies that made him laugh—a real "belly" laugh. As he recovered from his so-called "incurable" illness. Cousins went on to tell others of the healing power of laughter and the positive chemical changes in the body in the book *Anatomy of an Illness as Perceived by the Patient.*

Pick Your Mood

If you aren't sure how you typically act and react in life situations, take our Bright Side/Dark Side Quiz to determine your category.

A Look on the Bright Side :)

:) When things go wrong, I know that everything will work out for the best.

:) I wake up expecting the day to go well.

:) If something negative happens, I think of it as a fluke and not a pattern.

:) I think the world is getting better than it was when I was young.

:) I look at half a glass of water as being half full.

:) I look at life's interruptions as challenges to conquer.

:) A problem is just another puzzle that has a solution.

:) I wake up with the expectation that this will be an amazing day.

A Look on the Dark Side :(

:(When things go wrong, I am not surprised. In fact, when things go right, I worry about what will happen next.

:(I expect to have problems and often I do.

:(The world is much worse now than when I was young.

:(I wake up at night and worry.

:(I look at half a glass of water as half empty.

:(I often feel anxious just waiting for a problem to occur.

:(I dread waking up, knowing that I have to face another difficult day.

:(Problems are thorns in my life that keep me from accomplishing my goals.

I can complain because rosebuds have thorns . . . or rejoice because the thorn bush has a rose! It's all up to me.

—Anonymous

Turn Stumbling Blocks into Stepping Stones

How did you score? If you chose mostly :), you already know that optimistic or positive thinking will carry you far in life, especially when life's interruptions hit. If you're a perpetual pessimist, choosing mostly the :(or seeing just the dark side of life, we're going to teach you some easy ways to lighten up :)! In doing so, you will get the age-deactivating benefit of an optimistic outlook that will help you to be happier, lower your risk for disease, and keep you feeling and looking young.

Hosts of scientific experiments have shown that in order to experience optimal health, you need to "put on a happy face." In one landmark study at UCLA, researchers linked pessimism with a faster decline of immune function in HIV-positive persons. A closely related 13-year study at the National Center for Health Statistics found that those who were pessimistic were one and one-half times likelier to die of heart disease than optimists even when other risk factors were taken into account.

When you add to a pessimistic personality the traits of cynicism and hostility, you have the perfect breeding ground for stress-aging. At the 1997 meeting of the American Psychological Association, a discussion was held about cynicism and other negative emotions. Dr. Steven Rogelberg, a professor at Bowling Green State University, reported that cynicism, like depression and anxiety, can cause stress hormones to flow into the bloodstream, which can damage the cells that comprise your immune system. As you learned in Chapter 1, a weakened immune system will eventually give in to disease and accelerated aging.

How Cynical Are You?

So what's wrong with being a little cynical? Plenty, say experts. Research indicates that not only is it offensive to friends and family, but cynicism can lead to health problems. To help you understand the components of a cynical personality, take the following test. Give yourself 1 point for every question with which you strongly agree, 2 points if you slightly agree, 3 points if you slightly disagree, and 4 points if you strongly disagree.

_____ 1. Most people will tell a lie if they can gain from it.
_____ 2. People claim to have ethical standards but few stick to them when money's at stake.

_____ 3. People try to act more like they care about one another than they really do.

_____ 4. It's sad to see an unselfish person in today's world because so many people will try to take advantage of them.

_____ 5. Most people are just out for themselves.

_____ 6. Most people dislike putting themselves out to help other people.

_____ 7. Most people are dishonest by nature.

How Did You Score?

7–9: A real hard-boiled cynic.

10–12: A bit cynical, but probably refer to yourself as a realist.

13–16: More wary than cynical.

17–21: Skeptical but some trust in others.

22–26: Eternal optimist.

27–28: Probably too idealistic for your own good.

Wait Your Turn, and Live Longer

Hang on! There is more to this theory of negative personality activating aging and disease. You have probably heard of the so-called Type A personality. These people are quite literally slaves to the clock—always in a hurry and seldom taking time out to enjoy life. Type A individuals are time-oriented and frequently speak very rapidly, and impatiently finish the sentences of those they are speaking to. Type A people may also be hostile. This is in marked contrast to the Type B personality, who is quite simply a non-Type A; he gets the work done but also takes time out to smell the roses (see Table 2.1).

Researchers initially concluded that it was the Type A individual who was most likely to succumb to a heart attack yet that is

Table 2.1 Personality Types and Susceptibility to Illness

Type	Traits	Susceptibility to Illness
Type A	Angry, hostile, driven (anger needed for disease risk)	Heart disease
Type B	Non-type A, moves slower takes time to "smell roses"	Less risk than "angry" type A
Type C	Passive, endures great personal pain, says yes when prefers to say no	Increased risk of some cancers, frequent infections
Type D	Negative, insecure, distressed	Increased risk of heart disease
Type T	Thrill-seeking personality	Decreased life expectancy due to risks they take

only partly true. Scientists now know that it is not so much the time orientation that is responsible for the associated heart problems but rather the emotions associated with stress. The emotions of anger and hostility are critical due to the effect on stress and stress hormones. New studies show that the accumulation of these hormones is thought to make blood vessels more likely to constrict and may accelerate the formation of new blockages. Mark Goodman, a specialist in behavioral medicine, found that a Type A personality produced twice the likelihood that a patient would need to undergo a repeat angioplasty than calmer patients. Goodman found that personality type, and particularly the trait of hostility, were associated with arteries blocking again even after treatment with angioplasty. Post-surgery treatment in the clinic where the study was conducted now includes helping patients lessen their hostility to reduce the progression of artery blockage and the need for repeat surgery. Other personality types such as C, D, or T have also been linked to risk of disease or decreased life expectancy.

Anatomy 101

There is no such thing as a "pure" type A, B, C, D, or T personality. While it is true that our genetic code and early experiences can have a profound impact on our ultimate personality, the environment in which we find ourselves is equally important, and you might be a composite of all these personalities. It does turn out, though, that most of the time you will exhibit the characteristics of one or just a couple of these personality constructs.

Take a Chill Pill, and Call Me in the Morning

"Well, at least I'm not at high risk for a heart attack. I'm not angry, cynical, or even hostile. Most of the time, I'm in control. The only time I completely lose it is when I'm driving the interstate in morning rush hour traffic. Don't even think of cutting in front of me, or I will get you back!" Rob seemed like such a laid back guy that it was difficult to imagine him going berserk on the freeway. But if what he says is true, this is one negative behavior he may want to change—quickly.

A key marker for hostility in today's world is road rage, which is characterized by aggressive driving and the stress associated with getting stuck in traffic. Driving aggressively is not only dangerous but research suggests an association with heart disease risk because of its relationship to hostility in general. We find it curious how differently people react to this type of stress. Many tell of being like Rob, pumped up for battle as soon as they hit the crowded highways, daring another driver to make a false move. Yet others, like our good friend Ellen, actually enjoy getting stuck in traffic. Ellen writes letters, listens to music, sings, makes phone calls, and just generally has a good time. Ironically, Ellen says the most fun is watching the guy (probably Rob!) in the next car, slamming on the brakes, his knuckles white on the steering wheel, and cursing every few minutes.

Where Do You Turn for Comfort?

If hostility, cynicism, and a negative outlook on life all activate stress-aging, then where do we turn when life gets tough? While we have no control over most of life's stressors, there are some things we can control, and research is finding an important connection between longevity and social support. This support includes family, neighbors, and friends who help you to do the business of everyday life. A host of comprehensive studies now reveal that people who have strong social support tend to do better in every life situation, and that means less stress-aging.

"Get involved with more people? No way! I love spending time alone," Marny, a single parent, told us. "My sweet abode is my cocoon; my shelter from the harried world. In fact, after a stressful week of dealing with clients at work and my two daughters at home, I long for those quiet nights when I finally deadbolt the doors and protect my body from the intrusions of life. My motto? Call me a homebody . . . but please don't call me!"

Marny is not alone. Cocooning is epidemic today. But have we created such a rat race in our society that the only way we can cope is to hide? Ironically, while we say we want an island of sanity or peace, we are still obsessed with staying connected— just not in person. That's why millions have at their disposal several telephones, cellular phones, beepers, faxes, and computers to connect us to strangers on the Internet—just so we don't feel so alone. Does this make sense? Maybe. Keep reading!

Only give up a thing when you want some other condition so much that the thing no longer has any attraction for you, or when it seems to interfere with that which is more greatly desired.

—Gandhi

Perhaps our desire to reconnect with people—even strangers over the Internet—is an important reason for the growing quest for spirituality in our transient society. In years past, people lived close to family members and relied on parents and siblings for affirmation and emotional strength, even after marriage. When suffering occurred, people could turn to relatives for comfort and support. But with our highly mobile society, many adults today live hundreds of miles away from parents and siblings.

Why is this connection with others or social support so important? Close relationships with family and friends allow us to nourish our hungry souls. When we are tied emotionally to those we love, we can let out our feelings of fear, insecurity, and guilt and receive comfort from people who accept us—just as we are—with no strings attached. But if we have no place that feels safe enough to let down our emotional defenses, then we tend to keep our guard up all the time—a negative, cynical, and sometimes defensive guard that numbly masks the very problems we are facing.

Making Your Circle of Ten

Conditioned as we are to live as independent beings, the reality of deactivating stress-aging and staying young is "you gotta have friends." In that regard, how's your Circle of Ten? That means ten close connections—family, coworkers, neighbors, friends, or pets. We call this group our teammates.

Count your teammates, starting with family members with whom you have a close relationship—the ones with whom you share feelings, worries, and day-to-day events at least once a week. Then add up your friends and pets, and see how many are on your team.

1. _____ 6. _____
2. _____ 7. _____
3. _____ 8. _____
4. _____ 9. _____
5. _____ 10. _____

If your Circle of Ten is more like a Semicircle of Five, we will help you to expand the number as you start the EAT Plan (see Age Deactivator 2). We will teach you ways to increase your social support by narrowing down the types of professional, civic, or hobby groups you may enjoy, by giving tips on how to connect with a church or religious organization, and helping you find meaningful volunteer commitments that will benefit others as well as your immune system. You will find that the more you get out of your cocoon and start actively being with people, the less negative you will feel and the more apt you are to stop stress-aging.

In your Circle of Ten, we want you to identify one relationship that is special and intimate whether it is your spouse, your partner, or a special friend. A 5-year study at Duke University Medical Center found that unmarried heart disease patients who did not have a confidant were three times more likely to die early from cardiac disease than those who were married or had a close friend. Similar findings came in a Canadian study of 224 women with breast cancer. Seven years after diagnosis, 72 percent of the women with at least one intimate relationship survived; only 56 percent of those who did not have a confidant survived. The kind

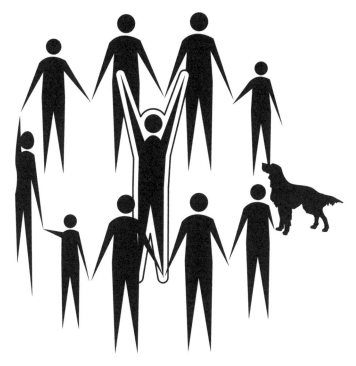

Figure 2.1

of intimacy necessary appears to be an emotional connection to someone, not necessarily a sexual relationship.

Just the Facts

Having an intimate relationship helps people feel cared for, helps maintain optimism, and aids in stress management. All of these emotional benefits lead to stronger immunity to help fight disease and stress-aging.

The benefits of intimacy extend beyond cancer and heart disease. In a nine-year study, California researchers examined the health of 7,000 Alameda County residents. They found that independent of all other risk factors—including smoking, drinking, and weight—loners faced a much greater risk of dying from all causes than did those with close ties to friends and family. In the *Journal of the American Medical Association,* Dr. Sheldon Cohen, a researcher at Carnegie Mellon University, reported that people with diverse social ties have a greater resistance to upper respiratory illness or colds; the more types of social ties, the more resistance to common colds and fewer cold symptoms.

Take a Tip from Joan of Arc

No, we're not asking you to die for something you passionately believe in, but there is another key ingredient of "soul food" that is vital to deactivating stress-aging, and this is having a sense of purpose and meaning for your life. For many people, this comes from having a spiritual or religious perspective. Others may be passionate about their work, their family, a goal, or a cause. Important elements of purpose and meaning in life include your level of faith and hope about the future, your system of beliefs, your ability to forgive and be connected to others, or the use of spiritual practices like meditation or prayer.

"See, I told you this was a religious plan!" Remember Jake? He kept trying to figure out the basis for the EAT Plan before we even finished the first part of our seminar. No, Jake, it's not about religion, but we are going to take a healing hint from some spiritual disciplines in order to experience reduced stress in the body.

As you learned on page 16, Dr. Herbert Benson of Harvard Medical School was one of the first medical researchers to study the interplay between the mind and body, specifically, the health benefits of prayer or meditation. Interestingly, Benson found that the exact words said in prayer are not important; all of the prayers

Table 2.2 The Relaxation Response

The relaxation response slows down the sympathetic nervous system, leading to:
  Decreased heart rate
  Decreased blood pressure
  Decreased sweat production
  Decreased oxygen consumption
  Decreased catacholamine production (brain chemicals associated
    with the stress response)
  Decreased cortisol production (stress hormone)

or meditations he tested resulted in healthful physiological changes. Remember in Chapter 1, we talked about stress and the fight-or-flight response? Well, according to Benson's studies, prayer leads to healthy changes known as the relaxation response, which brings about the opposite of fight or flight, helping to decrease cortisol secretion so optimal immune function can be restored.

Just the Facts
  Transcendental Meditation (TM) is a type of relaxation technique in which you sit comfortably with eyes closed and mentally repeat a Sanskrit word or sound (mantra) for 15 to 20 minutes, twice a day. It has been reported to help people think more clearly, improve their memory, recover from stress, reverse the aging process, and appreciate life more fully. In a study reported in the journal *Hypertension* (1996), TM was found to surpass other forms of relaxation therapies at lowering blood pressure. In this study, 111 African-American men and women, ages 55 to 85, were assigned to practice TM daily. The blood pressure reductions they experienced were similar to those commonly achieved with antihypertensive medicines. In long-term drug studies, such reductions have been associated with about 35 percent fewer strokes and heart attacks.

Together in Spirit

And—let's not forget to mention that those of you who are actively involved in some type of organized religion are well on your way to optimal health, according to ground-breaking scientific research. Two recent independent studies correlate greater attendance at religious services with increased physical health and longevity. The first study, published in October 1997 by Duke University Medical Center, involved more than 1,700 adults over age 65 in North Carolina. Those who attended church at least once a week were much less likely to have high levels of interleukin-6, an immune system protein associated with increased age-related disease. They also were less likely to have some cancers, autoimmune disorders, and certain viral diseases. Even doing everyday tasks such as walking, dressing, and cooking came easier to those who attended church.

The second study, in November 1997, was coauthored by researchers at Yale and Rutgers and followed 2,912 senior adults over a 12-year period. Those attending monthly religious services had better mental health, and were also less likely to smoke or consume alcohol. Even those who described themselves as chronically ill reported greater feelings of optimism and fewer symptoms of depression than those who did not attend at least monthly. It is not that healthy people simply attended services more often. In fact, many of the participants in both studies had severe disabilities. In the Rutgers study, there was evidence that attendance at religious services had a positive impact on health even after variables such as friendship, leisure activities, and social support were controlled. Dr. Harold Koenig, author of the Duke study, suggested that immune function is enhanced by feelings of togetherness and the experience of worship; that religious beliefs provide a worldview in which illness, suffering, and death can be better accepted or understood. Another explanation is that religious beliefs provide a self-esteem that is more lasting than other sources of self-esteem, such as material things, the way you look, or your physical abilities. All of these may change with increasing age and worsening health.

Real Food for the Soul

So, how can all of these issues fit together? How about at meal time, at the family dinner table? The American Dietetic Association Nutrition Trends Survey of 1997 reports that 28 percent of us skip meals very often or quite a bit, up from 21 percent in 1995. And 32 percent report eating out frequently. How often do you gather with family and friends for the evening meal? How often does your dining experience involve laughter, conversation, camaraderie, and enjoyment of eating?

A Personal Note

When Cathy visited Italy last year, she was intrigued to find that eating is such a priority that entire cities seem to shut down during meal time. In this European country, meal time is taken seriously with several food and wine courses; conversation and togetherness abound. Even decision-making business lunches are different. In Rome, Cathy observed a group of six businessmen who arrived at the restaurant on their bicycles, ordered a pitcher of Chianti, then feasted on hot, steaming pasta smothered in tomato-basil sauce with a side order of steamed spinach. This festive lunch was a lively two-hour affair with laughter interspersed between discussions of business. What a healthy way to spend the lunch hour and to accomplish the business of the day!

What about in your life? Do you make time to really enjoy the dining moment, or do you have a "grab it and go" mentality? Most of us treat meal time like we do all other areas of our lives—as one more obligation. We eat with the television on, the telephone ringing, and everyone in a hurry to get to the next item on their "To Do" list. As you will learn in the EAT Plan, even if you and your family can only manage a real "together meal" once a week, the value of slowing down and enjoying each other and the food in an atmosphere of lighthearted togetherness has to be good for the immunity.

Lighten Your Load

Let's face it. No matter what your age or life goal, growing older is tough enough without carrying a lot of excess emotional baggage. While there is no set remedy to look and feel young again, taking advantage of "soul food" is one proven way to give balance and emotional healing to your life, and the tools are right at your disposal.

As you will see in the EAT Plan, many components are crucial to stop stress-aging, and all of these work together to rejuvenate you. In the next chapter, we'll look at real food, and its role in staying healthy and young. We know that as you get in touch with your spiritual side, feed your body healing nutrients, and experience connectedness between body and soul, you can successfully get in control of stress-aging.

Chapter 3

Food, Your "Stay Young" Prescription

If you suffer from the ill effects of stress-aging, the saying "You are what you eat" is nothing new, as Mary Ann would testify. This 50-year-old single parent and editor of a popular woman's magazine claims to know all about the relationship between food and stress-aging, yet ignores this knowledge when it comes to her own health.

"Stress-aging? I'm living proof that it will sneak up on you and zap you of your energy and youthful good looks," Mary Ann told us a few months ago during a magazine interview. Her story is not uncommon and one you may relate to: a tumultuous relationship that ended in divorce, a rebellious teenager, two biopsies for precancerous conditions, a bone density test which revealed early stages of osteoporosis, and now a diet of black coffee to keep her alert followed by antacids because of an uncontrolled gnawing feeling in her stomach. While she writes a magazine food column, Mary Ann cannot remember the last time she personally focused on a healthy diet, and added, "My eating habits are so horrible that I wouldn't know how to cook broccoli

even if I bought some. If it doesn't come already prepared and
ready-to-serve, I don't eat it.''

Anatomy 101

Osteoporosis is thinning of the bones—a decrease in the
density of bones. It is not a natural sign of aging and can be
prevented with a diet high in calcium, weight-bearing exercises
such as walking or aerobics, taking estrogen at menopause (for
women), and using new bone-building medications, if recommended by your doctor. Understanding the stages of osteoporosis will enable you to see how bone loss and physical changes
occur over time.

- **Stage 1** usually begins after age 30 to 35. There are no
  symptoms, no signs, and no detection using bone density
  tests. Bone removal begins to outpace bone formation.
- **Stage 2** usually occurs after age 35. While there are no
  symptoms and no signs, detection is now possible using
  bone density tests.
- **Stage 3** usually occurs after age 45. At this stage, bones
  have become thin enough to result in fractures. Detection
  can still be made using bone density tests.
- **Stage 4** occurs at age 55 and older. Not only will you have
  more fractures, but pain and deformity may now result.
  Detection is made through X-rays and bone density tests.

Stress-Aging: The Silent Thief

If you are reading this book, you're probably already familiar
with stress-aging and the health problems that can suddenly creep
up on you. Maybe it started with a relationship problem that led
to sudden weight loss and poor eating habits. Or perhaps it began
with a new job or move to a new city, when in all your busyness,
you neglected your diet and experienced the effect of ill health.
Whatever the problem, we are here to tell you that food—scrump-

tious and nutritious healing food—is one part of the EAT Plan that you can easily add to your daily lifestyle, and it will make a difference in how you look and feel.

Lucky for her, Mary Ann has started to work on getting in control of stress-aging before it created further havoc with her health and productivity. Because of cutting edge research on food and aging, she is now convinced that nutrients do make a difference (and has subsequently learned how to cook broccoli three different ways!).

Conditioned though we are to think that aging is something that just "happens," in the past decade scientists have changed this perception. Breakthrough studies strongly demonstrate the tie between nutrition and a healthy immune system, and as nutritionists, we couldn't be more pleased. Deficiencies of single nutrients can result in altered immune responses which have been observed even when the deficiency is relatively mild.

As researchers turn out study after study linking stress with aging, we are more convinced than ever before that we can take control of that 70 percent of aging—the percentage that is not genetic but dominated by the way we live our lives (see Figure 3.1). That's the main reason we are convinced the EAT Plan is the optimal answer to staying young.

Because of the media hype, you are probably aware of the need for folic acid to prevent birth defects, calcium to keep osteoporosis at bay, and vitamin C to lessen the symptoms of a cold. But did you know that there are a host of nutrients and micronutrients that have an important influence on your immune response and subsequent wellness?

The New Vitamania

Based on scientific studies discussed in Chapter 1, we know that genetics probably determine the strength of your immune

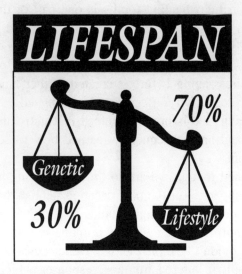

Figure 3.1

system. Nonetheless, there is mounting evidence that specific vitamins and minerals may be crucial for slowing down negative changes associated with aging. For example, vitamins A (beta-carotene), C, and E are known as antioxidants and are crucial antiaging nutrients. Zinc, selenium, folic acid, copper, iron, and magnesium are also involved in the formation of healthy new cells, including the white blood cells you need to fight off a host of potentially aging diseases and degenerative problems.

As such, each nutrient may play specific roles as *Immune Boosters—or Immune Busters.* Vitamin E is a major *Immune Booster* and may be aggressive against viral infections and respiratory illness, while zinc, another *Immune Booster,* fights against agents such as fungi, parasites, and viruses. Although the individual properties and functions of each nutrient are important, it is the sum of their effectiveness together that may really protect and strengthen the immune system and help stop stress-aging.

> **Just the Facts**
> Even when you suffer from a mild illness such as a common
> cold, nutrition is vital. Researchers have found that sucking on
> zinc gluconate lozenges at the start of a cold may lessen its
> severity. One study at Dartmouth College reported that students
> who took zinc lozenges at the onset of a cold had only five days
> of symptoms compared with nine days for students who received
> placebos. The theory is that zinc has an antiviral effect in the
> mouth and nose.

When Food Is Medicine

Every week, there is news about specific foods and their health
benefits. What is so special about these foods? Scientists have
studied them individually to try to determine their tie to longer
life.

Take the exotic kiwi. Data from Paul Lachance, Ph.D., a food
scientist at Rutgers, compared the delicate kiwi with other fruits
for nutrient density. Surprisingly, the kiwi had the highest nutrient
density for nine essential vitamins and minerals, followed by
papaya, mangoes, lemon, oranges, apricots, grapefruit, raspberries, strawberries, pineapple, plums, bananas, peaches, and apples.
In addition to nutrients like vitamins and minerals, kiwi is loaded
with antioxidants which are associated with slowing the aging
process and boosting the immune system changes we see with
stress.

Table 3.1 Antioxidant All-Stars

The USDA researchers analyzed the ability of common fruits and vegetables to act as antioxidants in the body. From highest to lowest, the best were:

1. Blueberries	6. Plums
2. Kale	7. Broccoli
3. Strawberries	8. Beets
4. Spinach	9. Oranges
5. Brussels sprouts	10. Red grapes

Just the Facts

If the ten fruits and vegetables listed are not among your favorites, try one of the runners up: red bell peppers, pink grapefruit, onions, white grapes, corn, eggplant, cauliflower, potatoes, cabbage, leaf lettuce, bananas, apples, green beans, carrots, tomatoes, and pears. Another study analyzing the antioxidant capability of fruit ranked from highest to lowest: strawberries, plum, orange, red grape, kiwi, pink grapefruit, white grape, banana, apple, tomato, pear, and honeydew melon.

And the Blue Ribbon Winner Is . . .

Why are blueberries the number one Antioxidant All-Star? The secret is in the color. The blue pigment *anthocyanin,* also found in strawberries and other blue-red fruits, is a potent antioxidant. A study by neuroscientist James Joseph of the U.S. Department of Agriculture reported that rats whose diets were supplemented with a few blueberries a day suffered fewer signs of the mental and physical slowing that can come with an aging brain. Diets with added strawberries and spinach were equally effective.

Lingo Lowdown

Resveratrol, a substance associated with reduced tumor growth and anticlotting effects similar to aspirin, is found in the skin of all red, green and blue-black grapes. These super age deactivators are also full of immune-boosting flavonoids.

Nuts to You

Another age deactivator is nuts, specifically, walnuts and peanuts. Researchers reported in the *New England Journal of Medicine* that men who included walnuts in their diet saw decreased serum cholesterol and favorable changes in other lipid levels as well as reduced blood pressure. Peanuts were found to contain resveratrol, the same antioxidant found in grapes and wine.

While you are writing down all of the new foods that can stop stress-aging, add avocados to your list. This nutrient-dense food has the highest fiber content of any fruit. Eating avocados will increase the antioxidant vitamins C and E, folate, potassium, and fiber in your diet; they are also free of saturated fat and cholesterol.

What Are Phytochemicals and Where Do I Get Them?

Scientists have identified chemical compounds within each of these foods that provide specific health benefits. These compounds are called *phytochemicals.*

Lingo Lowdown

Phytochemicals are biologically active substances that give plants their color, flavor, odor, and protection against disease. Some phytochemicals work as potent antioxidants. Antioxidants neutralize free radicals which have been associated with aging and many diseases from cataracts to cancer.

Let's look at the phytochemicals that have been identified in food groups and their tie to longer, healthier life.

Table 3.2 Power-Packed Phytochemicals

Phytochemical	Sources	How It Works
Fruits		
Limonene	Citrus fruits	Increases enzymes that break down carcinogens. Stimulates cancer-killing immune cells.
Ellagic acid	Grapes, apples, strawberries, raspberries	Slows tumor growth by decreasing enzymes used by cancer cells. May prevent carcinogens from damaging a cell's DNA, the first step in cancer development.
Anthocyanin	Blueberries, cranberries	Inhibits the production of proanthocyanin, a prostaglandin that can cause blood clotting.
Bioflavonoids	Red grapes, strawberries, bilberries, citrus fruits	Help the body dispose of potential cancer-causing chemicals, prevent free radical damage to eye tissue.
Orange, Red, and Dark Green Vegetables and Fruits		
Alpha-carotene	Pumpkin, carrots, cantaloupe, kale, yellow corn, seaweed	Slows the growth of cancer cells. May reduce risk of lung cancer and boost immunity.

Phytochemical	Sources	How It Works
Beta-carotene	Sweet potatoes, carrots, pumpkin, cantaloupe, apricots, peaches, spinach, leafy greens	Functions as an antioxidant, protects cells from free radical damage. May reduce risk of heart disease, bladder, colon, and skin cancer, boosts immunity.
Lycopene	Watermelons, tomatoes, tomato-based products, guava, pink grapefruit	Functions as an antioxidant, protects cells from free radical damage. May reduce risk of cardiovascular disease, colon, pancreatic, and prostate cancer.
Lutein and zeaxanthin	Kale, spinach, beets, collards, mustard greens, sweet red peppers	Function as antioxidants, protect cells from free radical damage. Filter out damaging light in the eye to reduce risk of macular degeneration. May reduce risk of lung, colon, and prostate cancer and boost immunity.
Capsaicin	Chili peppers	Prevents carcinogens like nitrates or cigarette smoke from getting through cell membranes. May also kill bacteria associated with ulcers. Increases circulation and may reduce risk of lung and other cancers.
Catechin flavonoid	Green tea	Functions as an antioxidant, protects

Phytochemical	Sources	How It Works
		cells from free radical damage, prevents platelets from sticking together. May reduce the risk of stomach, liver, and lung cancer and lower cholesterol levels.

Cruciferous Vegetables

Phytochemical	Sources	How It Works
Indoles	Broccoli, bok choy, cabbage, Brussels sprouts, cauliflower, kale, collards, kohlrabi, mustard greens, radishes, rutabaga, turnip greens, and turnips	Stimulate enzymes that make estrogen less active, improve immune response.
Isothiocyanates	Same as above	Increase enzymes that block carcinogens from cells, may slow tumor growth and reduce risk of lung cancer.
Sulforaphane	Same as above	Activates the liver to make enzymes that bind to carcinogens and transport them out of cells, suppresses tumor growth in animals.

Root Vegetables

Phytochemical	Sources	How It Works
Gingerol	Ginger root	Protects the stomach lining, prevents ulcer formation, stimulates gastric activity, stimulates the gall bladder, helps alleviate nausea.

Phytochemical	*Sources*	*How It Works*
Glycyrrhizin	Dried licorice root	Prevents testosterone conversion to potent form that may promote prostate cancer growth, stimulates the production of liver enzymes that reduce estrogen levels.
Allyl sulfide	Garlic or garlic supplements, onions, scallions, leeks, and chives	Increases enzymes that break down potential carcinogens and make them easier to excrete. May decrease the risk of stomach and colon cancer, lower LDL cholesterol levels. Improves immune response.

Beans and Grains

Genistein	Soybeans and soy products, peanuts, mung beans, and alfalfa sprouts	Blocks enzymes that switch on cancer genes, inhibits the growth of new blood vessels needed for tumor growth, blocks entry of estrogen into cells and testosterone into the prostate. Protects against breast cancer and prostate cancer. In lab studies, protects against all types of cancer cells including breast, colon, lung, prostate, skin, and leukemia. Other compounds in soy may reduce blood cholesterol levels.

Phytochemical	Sources	How It Works
Phytosterols, saponins	Soybeans, dried beans	Suppress the growth of cancer cells in the large intestine and enhance immunity.
Protease inhibitors	Soybeans, dried beans	Prevent the conversion of normal cells to cancer cells and slow tumor growth.
Phytic acid	Grains such as oats, rice, rye, and wheat, soybeans, peanuts, and sesame seeds	Prevents iron from producing cancer–causing free radicals, May reduce the risk of colon cancer.

Red Flag

What about *Immune Busters* such as saturated fats and trans-fatty acids? A diet high in saturated fats (found in meat and dairy products) and trans-fatty acids (found in margarine, snack and fast-food products, crackers, pastries, and many processed foods) can lead to many types of cancer, obesity, and even heart disease. According to findings at the Harvard School of Public Health reported in *The New England Journal of Medicine* (1998), women who eat diets high in saturated fat and trans-fatty acids were more likely to develop heart disease than women who consumed less of these fats. The researchers estimated that replacing 5 percent of total daily calories from saturated fat with unsaturated fat could reduce a woman's risk of heart disease by 42 percent. And replacing 2 percent of daily calories from trans-fatty acids with unhydrogenated, unsaturated fat (such as olive oil or canola oil) may reduce a woman's risk of heart disease by an estimated 53 percent.

Hey, What's Up, Doc?

"That's fine in theory. But when I get home at eight P.M. after an editorial meeting, I go by what's easiest to prepare, not the foods that are needed to stop stress-aging." While Mary Ann fully understood the healthy impact of nutrients in the body, she was painfully honest about how difficult it was to put this into practice. She told of good intentions to eat right, buying carrots, cabbage, and spinach at the grocery store, but opting instead for a small serving of canned green beans—simply because it was "quick and easy."

Mary Ann's seemingly vast knowledge of healthy eating combined with her less-than-healthy actions may seem contradictory, yet they are very common. The American Dietetic Association 1997 Nutrition Trends Survey reports that Americans do understand the impact of certain foods and food groups on health (see Table 3.3). But here's the catch: Although fruits and vegetables were named by 98 percent of those surveyed as contributing to health, we are not eating them! The USDA recently analyzed the top ten foods in America based on consumption, meaning what we actually eat (Table 3.4).

Isn't it interesting that with all the information on the importance of a low-fat, healthy diet, whole milk, soft drinks, and margarine contributed the most calories? Notice that there is not one fruit or vegetable on the list! A *USA Today* survey in May 1996 reported that the favorite vegetables of most adults were broccoli (19.7 percent), corn (15.1 percent), beans (11.9 percent), carrots (10.8 percent), and potatoes (8.8 percent). But this apparently doesn't translate into eating those veggies.

Table 3.3
Impact of Food Groups on Overall Health

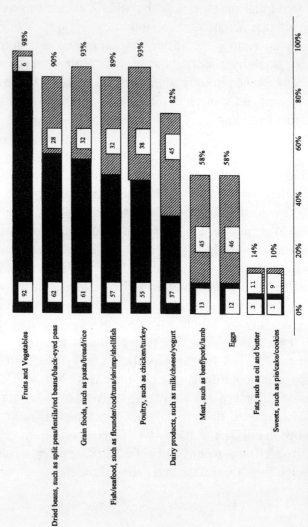

■ **Very Healthy Effect** ▨ **Somewhat Healthy Effect**

Fruits and Vegetables	92 / 6	98%
Dried beans, such as split peas/lentils/red beans/black-eyed peas	62 / 28	90%
Grain foods, such as pasta/bread/rice	61 / 32	93%
Fish/seafood, such as flounder/cod/tuna/shrimp/shellfish	57 / 32	89%
Poultry, such as chicken/turkey	55 / 38	93%
Dairy products, such as milk/cheese/yogurt	37 / 45	82%
Meat, such as beef/pork/lamb	13 / 45	58%
Eggs	12 / 46	58%
Fats, such as oil and butter	3 / 11	14%
Sweets, such as pie/cake/cookies	1 / 9	10%

0% 20% 40% 60% 80% 100%

The American Dietetic Association Nutrition Trends Survey, 1997.

Table 3.4 USDA Survey Top Ten Foods in America

1. Whole milk	6. Rolls and buns
2. Soft drinks	7. White flour
3. Margarine	8. White bread
4. Sugar	9. American cheese
5. Low-fat milk	10. Ground beef

How Much Is Enough?

The USDA has recommended that Americans get five fruit and vegetable servings a day. The serving size is small, only one-half cup. Yet only about 22 percent of all Americans eat the recommended five servings a day. States with the most five-a-day eaters (above 30 percent) include: Connecticut, Kansas, Massachusetts, Michigan, and New Jersey. States with the fewest (less than 19 percent) include: Alaska, Delaware, Iowa, Kentucky, Mississippi, North Carolina, North Dakota, and Utah. Interestingly, while adults are not taking advantage of immune-boosting fruits and vegetables, neither are their children! The proportion of high schoolers who ate at least five-a-day doubled between 1993 and 1995, but only rose from 14 percent to 28 percent.

Why do we share all this information? Because the nutrients found in the foods you eat are just as important as "soul food." Not only must you feed your inner spirit, but you must feed your body to stop stress-aging. A study in the *British Medical Journal* reported that diets that include plenty of fresh fruits, vegetables, and grains can help people prolong their lives. People who ate fresh fruits every day were 24 percent less likely to die from heart disease and 32 percent less likely to die of stroke than those who ate fresh fruit less often. About 40 percent of the population living the longest were vegetarians.

Table 3.5

HOW IMPORTANT ARE DIET AND NUTRITION TO YOU PERSONALLY?

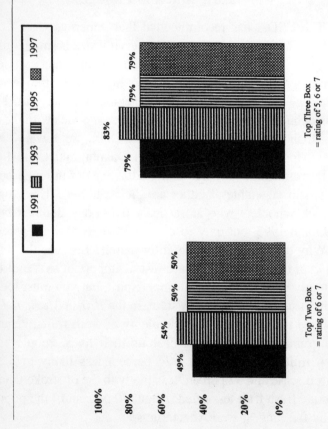

The American Dietetic Association Nutrition Trends Survey, 1997.

Just the Facts

One benefit of a diet high in fruits and vegetables may be lower blood pressure. In the study financed by the National Heart, Lung and Blood Institute known as DASH (Dietary Approaches to Stop Hypertension), participants ate a diet low in fat (less than 30 percent of daily calories), and high in fruits and vegetables (8 to 10 servings a day) and grains (7 to 8 servings). At the end of the study, the systolic blood pressure readings (the top number) dropped an average of 11 points. The diastolic pressure (the bottom number) dropped more than 5 points.

Americans realize the importance of diet and nutrition as reported by The American Dietetic Association 1997 Trends Survey (Table 3.2). In 1997, 50% rated diet and nutrition in their top two issues important to health and 79% rated them in their top three. But only 39% say they are doing all they can to eat healthfully.

Veggin' Out

"I'd be a vegetarian if my family would go along. Broccoli, kale, cauliflower—these are my favorite foods, but my husband and son will only eat green peas and corn." Maria could not understand why she loved the taste of strong-flavored vegetables yet her family could not bear to smell them cooking. It may not be in their heads, Maria!

One group who may shy away from eating the recommended fruits and vegetables are a group known to researchers as *supertasters*. These are people who have more taste buds and seem to be specifically sensitive to bitter tastes. Dr. Adam Drewnowski, at the University of Washington, reported in the *American*

Journal of Clinical Nutrition that supertasters tend to dislike the taste of *naringin,* a cancer fighter found in grapefruit juice. Other foods that are bitter may be totally offensive to them.

Anatomy 101
Who is a Supertaster?
To find out if you are a supertaster, Drewnowski recommends painting your tongue with a cotton tip dipped in blue food coloring. If it's mostly blue with occasional pink dots, you're a normal taster. If you see many big pink taste buds grouped closely together, chances are you are a supertaster and are prone to dislike broccoli, spinach, or kale. Supertasters can substitute the sweeter deep red and deep orange vegetables such as beets, carrots, squash, or pumpkin for those that taste bitter.

Eat Less and Live Longer

"I've heard about calorie restriction and longevity. Is that really the answer? I can't even eat the minimum calories recommended for women without being hungry. How can I cut back even further?" These are very common questions that we hear at most seminars.

Two new studies add to the evidence that supports eating less to live longer. The first study was done on monkeys and was published in the *American Journal of Physiology.* Researchers found that a 30 percent reduction in calories led to higher HDL levels, lower triglyceride levels, and a drop in blood pressure. The second study published in the *Journal of Clinical Endocrinology and Metabolism* showed that caloric reduction in monkeys helped slow down the body's natural decrease in the level of the hormone DHEA, one of the indicators of aging seen in humans. These researchers concluded that nutritional intervention has the potential to alter aspects of aging in long-lived species such as monkeys and humans.

The problem of the "eat less and live longer" theory is that, for many of us, it is difficult to cut back further on calories. I mean, can we really eat 30 percent fewer calories than we do right now? Or would the calorie restriction be so severe you would rather not live longer? We have given serious consideration to ways calories can be reduced without experiencing feelings of deprivation, and in the EAT Plan, we'll give some easy ways to cut unnecessary calories without giving up taste, enjoyment, and the benefits to health associated with many foods.

Recommended Dietary Allowances May Not Be Enough

The Food and Nutrition Board of the National Academy of Sciences issues Recommended Dietary Allowances (RDAs) for vitamins and minerals; these are the levels of nutrients thought to be adequate to meet the known nutrient needs of most healthy individuals. This means that the RDAs will help to prevent deficiency-related diseases such as beriberi or scurvy—diseases that are probably not on your list of concerns right now! Yet the RDAs that are sufficient for normal growth and prevention of nutritional deficiencies are frequently much lower than the amounts associated in the research with improved immunity or cancer prevention.

While we encourage you to increase your consumption of fruits and vegetables you may well need supplements of antioxidants, as shown in Table 3.5, to obtain the levels that offered protection in human and animal studies.

Table 3.5 Age-Deactivating Supplements

- Vitamin C: 250–500 mg daily
- Vitamin E: 200–400 IU daily
- Multivitamin and mineral supplement daily
- Calcium: Food sources or supplement to equal 1,000–1,500 mg daily

---

Just the Facts
We recommend checking out the "silver" and "over 50" multivitamin and mineral formulas because the mineral levels are more appropriate for most people, whatever their age. Additional mineral supplements can be added in special cases.

The Herbal Medicine Cabinet

Not only are studies confirming that food can help heal the body and stop stress-aging, but alternative medicine and herbal and related products to boost immunity are becoming increasingly popular. Although some of these products have been promoted as panaceas with little scientific data to support their use, clinical data are accumulating that show the benefit of specific herbs (see Table 3.6). In fact, even the National Institutes of Health (NIH) has turned its head "cautiously" toward alternative treatments such as herbs to sort out the truth from the hype. The NIH's Office of Alternative Medicine is funding studies aimed at establishing or disproving the clinical basis of different types of alternative therapy. While this marks a step in the right direction, the amount of money being spent to research unconventional treatments is only about $14 million of the NIH's staggering $11 billion annual budget, perhaps not nearly enough to make a difference.

> **Red Flag**
> With more than 1,600 herbal products on the market, and more than $1.5 billion spent on herbal treatments annually, make sure you don't pay too much. Many herbs and supplements are available at national discount chain stores for half the price charged by a small health food store.

Buyer Beware

No matter what the advertising flyer claims at the natural food store, even the most popular herbal compounds have ingredients that have not been tested and are not scrutinized by the Food and Drug Administration (FDA). Just because something is natural does not mean that it is safe. Hemlock is a natural product—but deadly!

Here's the latest evidence on popular supplements and herbal therapies with immune-boosting claims:

Table 3.6 Popular Supplements and Herbal Therapies

Product	Dose	Benefit/Concerns
Echinacea	500–1,000 mg every 2 hours until symptoms improve. Reduce dose to 2–5 times daily for up to 1 week. For prevention of infections, may be used 2–3 times daily for 1–2 weeks per month. Continued use should not exceed 8 weeks.	Supportive therapy for colds and flu, respiratory infections, and lower urinary tract infections. Boosts immune response. Significant side effects have not been reported but allergies are a possibility. Echinacea is not recommended for patients with tuberculosis, multiple sclerosis, HIV, and autoimmune diseases.
Garlic	1–2 g fresh garlic cloves, 8 mg essential oil of garlic, ¼–½ tsp dried powder	Prevention and treatment of heart disease and hypertension. Side effects include heartburn,

Product	Dose	Benefit/Concerns
		flatulence, gastrointestinal distress, allergic reactions, asthmatic reactions with repeated exposure to garlic dust, and changes in the odor of skin and breath. May reduce clotting time of the blood and should not be used by persons taking aspirin or other anticoagulants.
Ginkgo	40–60 mg ginkgo biloba extract (GBE) 2–3 times daily for 6–8 weeks	Considered an immune-boosting antioxidant, for treatment of vertigo, improvement of vasodilation and blood flow in the brain; memory effects are unclear. Side effects include headache, GI upset, and dizziness. Large doses may cause restlessness, nausea, vomiting, and diarrhea. Clotting time of the blood is reduced so anticoagulant medication may be affected.

Red Flag

Herbs and medications do not mix. Ginkgo, garlic, ginger, ginseng, and white willow bark are all blood thinners. If taken with aspirin or anticoagulant drugs, they could cause excess bleeding or even a stroke.

Table 3.7 Coming Soon!

* Carrots with 3–5 times the beta-carotene of regular carrots
* Beets with more folic acid to help prevent heart attacks and strokes
* Cucumbers with orange flesh to provide beta-carotene
* Onions and leeks that contain more of a protein to make blood less likely to clot
* Strawberries with more ellagic acid for cancer prevention
* Condensed orange juice with the phytochemical content of many oranges
* Snack foods with cholesterol–lowering phytochemicals
* Cheddar cheese with added iron and no change in flavor
* Genetically altered soybeans that reduce oligosaccharides which can cause flatulence
* Calcium-fortified juices with other vitamins boosted (such as vitamin C)

Nutraceuticals: The New Fast Food

In addition to healthy foods and herbal remedies, the race is on for products that provide specific health benefits. With a population of more than 70 million aging baby boomers as well as an enormous increase in health awareness among all Americans, the marketplace is seeing an enormous increase in food products called *nutraceuticals* or *functional foods*. These are nutritional products that have reasonable scientific evidence supporting health benefits. Nutraceuticals fall under the regulatory umbrella of the Dietary Supplement and Health Education Act of 1994 (DSHEA). If a nutraceutical product meets the Food and Drug Administration's requirements it can use its health claims in its marketing. Nutraceutical products fall into broad categories including vitamin and mineral supplements, herbal products, food and beverage products, and sports nutrition products. (See Table 3.7 for a list of healing nutraceuticals coming soon to your neighborhood.)

Lingo Lowdown

The term "nutraceutical" means "food medicine." These are foods or food products that have specific nutrients or herbs added to them to provide a medicinal effect in the body.

While there are no specific "magic" foods that are proven to stop stress-aging, research continues to confirm that there are some positive nutritional measures you can take to heal your body from the ravages of stress. Eating healthful foods helps maximize energy, alertness, and productivity, while minimizing the constant fatigue and lethargy that accompany stress-aging.

As you continue reading Chapter 4 on the value of activity and exercise, remember that in order to stop stress-aging, you must find the balance of a sound body, mind, and spirit. Good health is more than just the absence of disease, and taking charge of the areas of your health that you can control helps to optimize how you look and feel, while stopping stress-aging in its tracks.

Chapter 4

Rev It Up!

There is no question about the value of exercise or movement for weight loss, heart disease prevention, or good health. But listen to this: The verdict is in that *exercise is also crucial to deactivate stress-aging.* Before you close the book and start running . . . in the opposite direction . . . why don't you give us a chance to explain? Not only have we seen the age-deactivating benefit of exercise in our personal lives, but assessing thousands of clients and seminar participants over the past 15 years has further confirmed the theory. Those who are physically active are more likely to stay healthy and look and feel younger than those who are not active at all.

"Yeah, yeah. I've heard it before," you might say. "Somehow knowing that exercise is the key to good health and staying young isn't enough to make me budge out of the chair." Sure, we know you are tired and harried, as many of us are these days. Who said life was easy? Perhaps the only activity you get is channel surfing while curled up in a fetal position in your leather recliner.

Well, it doesn't matter. No matter what shape you're in, the information in this chapter will definitely provide that extra boost you need to get out of that chair and move around more, and in doing so, help you stop stress-aging in its tracks. But first let's dispel some common misconceptions about exercise and its relationship to staying young.

Truth or Consequences

Look at the following myths about exercise, then read the *truth and proof* as to why exercise is crucial to deactivate stress-aging.

Myth: *Exercise makes me too tired to think clearly.*
Truth: Wrong! Stress overload makes you too tired to think clearly. Exercise helps to boost brain power.
Proof: Not only does exercise increase blood flow to the brain, clinical research suggests that moving around more helps the brain receive much-needed nutrients and oxygen. According to Robert Dustman, Ph.D., Director of the Neuropsychology Research Lab at the VA Medical Center in Salt Lake City, you may be in your sixties but exercise will keep your brain cranking like a 30-year-old's. Dustman concludes that the better shape you're in, the faster you fire brain waves that are responsible for the quick thinking normally associated with youth. Regular exercise also produces alpha waves in the brain, which are tied to the feeling of serenity and relaxation.

Not only can exercise help a blue mood but British researchers say it may also boost your creative ability. Scientists at Middlesex University in England compared the aerobic benefits of workouts or dance to watching videos. The exercise group fared better on creativity tests than the nonexercise group. You might say that exercise will give you that competitive edge over less active colleagues as you age.

> **Lingo Lowdown**
> Alpha waves are brain waves that are prominent during
> relaxed wakefulness.

Myth: *Too much exercise tears down the immune system and
causes me to get sick easily.*

Truth: Wrong! Exercise puts the gears of your immune system
into high speed. When you begin to exercise, your white blood
cells start to increase in number. After your workout, the number
and aggressiveness of certain immune cells such as NK (natural
killer) cells increases by as much as 50 to 300 percent. Regular
workouts can produce these results consistently. Although the
count returns to a normal level after a few hours, the temporary
increases may help to cull out intruders and make the immune
system more efficient at destroying these bad guys throughout
the day. When you work out consistently (without overexercising), your immune system becomes a powerful weapon against
flu, colds, and other infections.

Proof: In a comprehensive study that shed light on the importance of exercise for immune strength, David Nieman, Ph.D., a
health researcher at Appalachian State University, found that
women in their thirties who walked 5 days a week for about 45
minutes were ill only 5 days during the study period of 15 weeks.
Their sedentary peers were sick for 10 days during this time. He
later studied women in their sixties to eighties who walked about
37 minutes per day, 5 days a week, for 12 weeks and found that
50 percent of the nonexercisers caught colds and flu while only
21 percent of the walkers did. Researchers suggest that people
with chronic illnesses such as HIV may also benefit from regular,
moderate exercise.

A closely related study by Arthur LaPerriere, at the University
of Miami School of Medicine, yielded the same results. LaPerriere
found that the CD4 count of people infected with HIV increased

when they rode bikes 3 times a week for about 45 minutes. Nieman's studies indicate that the T-cell count of 65-year-olds who exercise regularly is as high as those of people in their thirties. Regular exercise seems to slow down this once considered inevitable decline in immune function.

Red Flag

Do you exercise when you have a cold? Exercise should not worsen your cold, but if you have symptoms such as fever, aches, vomiting, coughs, or diarrhea, you may want to slow down. Your body is telling you that it is stressed, and you would be better off temporarily curled up in your favorite blanket, sipping a mug of hot chicken soup.

Myth: *I believe that taking time out to relax more instead of moving around more will help me live longer. I'm in my mid-fifties and surely don't want to burn out!*

Truth: Wrong! Exercise and activity are the keys to increased longevity, no matter how old you are.

Proof: A recent article in *Journal of the American Medical Association (JAMA)* discussed a landmark study following more than 15,000 people from 1977 through 1994. In this experiment, researchers found that leisure time physical activity is associated with reduced death even after genetic and other family-related factors are taken into account. The results of a variety of studies suggest that if every American got up off the couch and walked for an hour per day, our country could save *$20 billion* in related health care costs.

Myth: *Exercise makes me overeat, causing weight gain.*

Truth: Not only will exercise help you reduce your stress load and keep you from binging on food, it will help you whittle down that expanding waistline.

Proof: Sophisticated research performed in Sweden suggests that stress may be related to obesity and to central fat deposits or abdominal fat (apple shape). Stress causes an increase in the production and release of cortisol, which may cause the buildup of fat in the inner tube area of our body. Per Bjorntorp, a researcher in the Department of Heart and Lung Diseases at Sahlgren's Hospital and the University of Göteborg, Sweden, looked at more than 1,000 men and found that negative stressors were associated with a higher waist to hip ratio. What is the great moderator of stress? That's right—exercise!

Just the Facts

Lawrence Golding, Ph.D., director of exercise physiology at the University of Nevada, Las Vegas, says that as we age, body fat doesn't have to increase nor flexibility and strength decrease. In fact, much of "aging" is due to just sitting around. His research compared participants who had been in his exercise class for twenty years with that of the normal population. His class had body fat averages of 20 percent compared with the average of 26 percent. In addition, regular stretching wiped out any loss of flexibility with age.

No Time for Excuses

If you want excuses for not exercising, we can give you some, for we have heard them all. Perhaps the greatest excuse we hear from both men and women is that there is *no time* to exercise. Connie, a 44-year-old nurse practitioner and single mother of four, laughed when we mentioned the importance of scheduling exercise on her daily calendar.

"Schedule time to exercise? Let's see, I get up at five A.M., so there's no time before work. I arrive at the hospital at six-thirty, then get home at six P.M., so the day is pretty full. I guess

I could tell the kids to get their own dinner, or I could wake up in the middle of the night to start jogging on the treadmill." Connie may not have had time, but she did have a great sense of humor and eventually learned how to fit exercise in her busy life. How? She joined a family softball team with her four children at their church. Last we heard, she had dropped 15 pounds, felt like a kid again, and was enjoying some new teammates in her Circle of Ten, as discussed in Chapter 2.

While you haven't seen these excuses on David Letterman's show—yet—check out the ten most common excuses we hear for why people don't exercise:

The Top Ten Reasons People Don't Exercise

1. "I'd rather die than do aerobics next to those buff younger women in the skimpy leotards."
2. "Too tired. I need to save my energy to be productive at work."
3. "No way! Since I hit thirty-five, it takes me twice as long to ride my bike half as far as I used to. Why bother?"
4. "Exercise leaves me feeling exhausted and achy. It's not a fun experience."
5. "To be honest, I'm allergic to sweat."
6. "The dog ate my tennis shoes (jogging pants, bathing suit, treadmill)."
7. "I fall asleep during exercise, so I have to avoid it for safety reasons."
8. "I read somewhere that the heart is programmed with only so many beats, and I'd sure hate to waste these on exercise."
9. "I ate my tennis shoes (jogging pants, bathing suit, treadmill)."
10. "I'm focusing on rewarding myself with life's simple

pleasures to find happiness. I'd rather eat (sleep, veg out, stare, daydream, watch TV) than exercise!''

Excuses. We've heard them all, from *"no time,"* to *"no energy,"* to *"no motivation."* But the honest truth is that *"no exercise"* is going to push stress-aging into high gear.

We know you are busy. *Who isn't?* We know it's difficult to find time to work out as often as you would like. *It's hard for everyone.* Nonetheless, the good news is that you can accumulate 30 minutes of vigorous movement throughout the day and still get great benefits—enough to deactivate stress-aging and activate those youthful good looks again.

No Matter What Gear (or Shape) You're In

How about it? Are you one of the smart ones, going full speed ahead, or have you been idling in neutral far too long? Take the following quiz to see what gear you're in, then we will tell you some surprising ways to rev yourself up and gain the benefit of deactivating stress-aging.

1. I have stairs at work or in my house, and I use them regularly.	___ Yes	___ No
2. I park farther away from where I am going on purpose.	___ Yes	___ No
3. I lift boxes or packages, and walk a lot at work.	___ Yes	___ No
4. I take care of my own laundry and housekeeping.	___ Yes	___ No
5. I walk or ride my bike to do errands when possible.	___ Yes	___ No
6. I do my own yard work and gardening.	___ Yes	___ No
7. I play active games with kids often.	___ Yes	___ No
8. My relaxation time is spent being active.	___ Yes	___ No

9. I try to exercise while watching television, especially during the commercials or the news. ___ Yes ___ No
10. I go to the gym or take a 30-minute walk five times during the week. ___ Yes ___ No

Guilty or Not?

If you answered "yes" to *six or more* of these statements, you probably get the 30 minutes a day of activity. We consider you *"not guilty"* of neglecting this vital Age Deactivator. Nevertheless, if you chose "no" at lease *five or more times,* then the verdict is in: *Guilty!* You have ignored engaging in enough movement and activity to stop stress-aging in its tracks, and your sentence is . . . *exercise!*

Oh, come on! It's never too late to get that engine out of idle and get those buns moving. Keep reading to learn how.

A Love Affair with Lethargy

We know you have friends who never seem tired, nor do they look tired or old. These same people have just as many commitments as you do—or even more—yet they are full of energy, enthusiasm, and life itself. Chances are these friends get regular exercise, for without it, weak, unexercised muscles poop out.

"Ah, so that's why I feel so lethargic? As little exercise as I get, my muscles are probably atrophied." Thirty-nine-year-old Seth's love affair with lethargy had made him look and feel ten years older, and while he made jokes about his shrinking muscles, this was no laughing matter. When Seth told our audience how his stair-stepper had turned into an efficient towel rack after one use, we knew he needed some extra motivation.

Seth, if you are reading this, we hope you took our advice to heart—literally! Your body is pleading for exercise (although you probably find this hard to believe). And since you are approaching forty, it's time to start working on the internal (heart, lungs, muscles, and joints) and external parts to stay fit and to reclaim those youthful good looks.

Now if you are like Seth and absolutely dread the word *exercise*—much less actually doing it—the good news is that exercise is loosely defined, meaning if your heart is pumping and calories are burning, chances are the activity can be classified as ''exercise.'' (Yes, sex does count as a calorie-burning, heart-pumping activity!)

Not only does exercise include jogging around the track, working out at the gym, or doing aerobics with a Jane Fonda lookalike, but there are a host of daily activities such as raking leaves, working in your garden, taking a brisk walk out-of-doors or at the mall, playing with the dog or kids, and mopping or vacuuming your house that qualify as well.

Lingo Lowdown
Exercise includes any physical activity that burns calories and makes your heart beat faster.

Common Daily Activities That Are Also Exercise

_____ Cleaning house	_____ Mopping Floors
_____ Climbing stairs	_____ Mowing the lawn
_____ Gardening	_____ Playing with children
_____ Lifting groceries	_____ Raking leaves
_____ Shopping at the mall	_____ Walking the dog

Keep the Dimples on Your Face

Dimples belong on your face, not on your backside! Here's some advice that will keep that gorgeous dimpled face of yours smiling at the next class reunion. Experts recommend that everyone burn off through activity about 1,400 calories per week, and gradually increase that number to 2,000+ calories per week. For example; if you expend 1,200 to 1,300 calories per week through walking, try to make up the 700 to 800 calorie difference by chasing the dog, playing with your children, lifting those bags of mulch for your garden, and quickly climbing the stairs at home or at the office.

To deactivate stress-aging, your goal is to burn *at least 200 calories* per day. You can accumulate your 200 calories throughout the day by going up and down stairs at work, walking to the deli several blocks from your office at lunch time, parking in the back of the lot when you stop at the grocery store after work, and carrying in those heavy bags of groceries. The next day, walk the mall like you mean it while looking for that birthday gift for your best friend. When you get home, take the dog out for a brisk walk around the neighborhood for some fresh air, give your car a once-over with a damp sponge—bend, reach, pull, turn, again and again—then finish your day with a quick vacuum throughout the house before dinner. Notice that we are talking about real-world exercise through daily living . . . the best way to stop stress-aging and look young.

Whatever you do, it's important to do activities or exercise you enjoy or you won't be doing them for very long. Studies show that the more enjoyable the activity, the more you will do it, the better you feel and look, the more weight you drop, the more energized your mind, and the stronger your heart (see Figure 4.1). Do you get the picture now?

CYCLE OF EXERCISE AND ACTIVITY

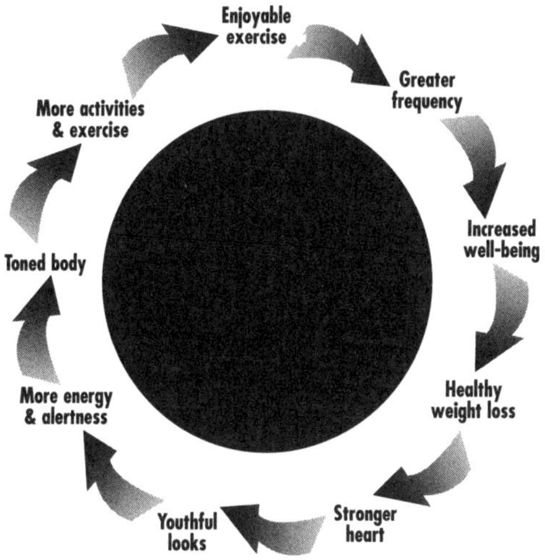

Figure 4.1. Cycle of Exercise and Activity

Get the Big Nip and Tuck . . . And It's Free!

"Cellulite and flab don't just run in my family. They gallop." Kim, a young electrical engineer for a large corporation, found that her new sedentary job combined with little exercise was leaving its mark on her body—a growing flabby mark on her thighs she did not want to wear.

Kim continued: "For as long as I can recall, every woman in my family at age thirty-five has stopped wearing shorts or a bathing suit because of gravity's increased pull on their hips and rows of dimpled cellulite on their thighs. Aunt Marianne even tried liposuction only to have the flab reappear one year later. Isn't there another alternative to the tug of gravity and the thigh dimples we all inherited?"

So, Kim, though you ignore all the "rules" of staying toned by sitting all day and avoiding exercise, you now want a magical concoction to make you look great and stop stress-aging? Perhaps you've been doing sedentary aerobics with the remote control for some time, and now that your wrist and fingers are supple and slim, it's time to focus on losing the dimples from your hindside. Well, we have just the elixir: weight training!

The more we assess the research, the more we are convinced that weight training is a main key to unleashing the answers to stress-aging. According to the federally funded "Women Across America" study, middle-aged women (ages 40 to 55) feel more aches and pains and are physically weaker than previously believed. This study confirms that women in this middle-age bracket often have significant difficulty climbing a flight of stairs, carrying groceries, or even walking around the block. Why? Because body composition changes as we age, and although you may weigh the same, you start to lose muscle and gain more body fat. This loss in muscle mass, known as *sarcopenia,* is a direct cause of decreased muscle strength. This muscle loss seems to start around age 25, although fat hides much of the loss for many years.

Experts say that from age 20 to 60, the average woman's body fat percentage will increase from 33 to 44 percent while a man will see an increase in body fat from 18 percent to 36 percent. Every 10 years, men and women both lose about 6.5 pounds of muscle. Where did it go? Well, don't look too hard now. All that muscle went by way of the television, elevator, car, computer, golf cart, and all the other modern-day miracles that don't require us to work quite as hard as our ancestors did.

Hope or Hype?

"Wait a minute. I said diminish the dimples and flatten the flab, not bulk me up like a body builder." Kim, the young woman who thought cellulite was a requirement for position on her family tree, was hesitant when we mentioned weight training to tighten up those sagging muscles. Like Kim, many women still associate weight training with building bulky muscles, but this is simply not true. Check out the following common misconceptions about weight lifting. Can you tell which is true and which is hype?

1. ***Weight lifting is dangerous.*** Hype. If done with proper technique, this is a very safe and effective way to tone the body and stay young.
2. ***If you stop, muscles will turn to fat.*** Hype. This is physiologically impossible. If you stop weight lifting, the muscles will lose size and tone, and any excess calories will be deposited as fat.
3. ***Women will get big muscles.*** Hype. Women produce less testosterone than men, and they also have 30-40% less muscle fiber.
4. ***Weight training means always using heavy equipment.*** Hype. Resistance bands can be used in weight training. Other ways to train include using isometrics, free weights or even water resistant exercises.
5. ***You must start with heavy weights.*** Hype. You should *not* begin with heavy weights. A good rule of thumb is to start with a weight you can easily lift 10 times with the last 2 repetitions being increasingly difficult. For some people this is only 1 to 2 pounds; others can start at 15 to 20 pounds or more, depending on their muscle strength. As your muscles gain strength and if there is no pain, increase the weights in 5- to 10-pound increments.
6. ***The theory "no pain, no gain" is true for strength training.*** Hype. If your muscles are very sore, do not use resistance training until you are relatively pain-free. Strength training may not be appropriate for everyone, so check with your doctor for approval.

7. **You will get high blood pressure.** Hype. Weight training does not cause high blood pressure. Some people strain their body and hold their breath during a lift, which results in a temporary increase of blood pressure. However, this is *never* recommended during weight training.

8. **You will become bulky and inflexible.** Hype. It is important to supplement your weight training with a stretching routine to stay flexible.

9. **Lifting weights helps me spot-reduce specific areas of my body.** Hype. Exercise is not site specific; you must exercise the total body to achieve maximum results.

10. **The benefits are many.** Totally true! Increased strength, improved muscle tone, enhanced athletic performance, increased bone strength, injury prevention, and improved body image are all benefits of weight training. For women, weight training can play a significant role in reducing osteoporosis, as bones need regular resistance to stay strong. And age is no factor with weight training; the muscles of older people are just as responsive as those of younger people.

And the Winner Is . . . Weight Training

Here's the case we plead for weight training, and we think it's a winner. Working your muscles with light weights or rubber bands (even cans of black beans or chicken soup from the pantry) will build lean muscle mass, which by the way makes your metabolism go faster. Weight training will also help to preserve the muscle mass you already have, tone your body, and get rid of a lot of those pesky aches and pains many associate with stress-aging. The exciting news is that experts suggest that you can *decrease your body fat by 1 to 2 percent every 4 to 6 weeks* until you approach your desired level. Now that is some Age Deactivator, isn't it?

Just the Facts
Fat burns 2 to 3 calories per pound while muscle burns 50 calories per pound.

Muscle mass is the metabolically active tissue. This means it's the tissue that burns calories. The more muscle mass your body has, the more calories you burn all day, every day, even while you are sitting around. Now you know why men seem to lose weight so much faster than women. They often have more muscle mass so they burn more calories.

A Personal Note

Susan was so impressed by all the research on weight training as an Age Deactivator that she decided to modify her regular aerobic exercise routine and add light weights 2 times a week. Two months before a trip to Germany, where she was going to be carrying a back pack and hauling luggage from trains to hotels, Susan started using 10-pound weights and doing a set of simple exercises at home. She now lifts weights (still light ones) twice a week for 30 minutes to an hour depending on her schedule. She is amazed at how toned she looks now, and her husband commented that she has more spring in her step.

We Want Results . . . Today

"I could clean out my bedroom closet or mop the entire house in the time it takes to do three sets of twelve exercises," Sarah said. Many of our friends think that weight training takes too long and even tag this "wait training." But this is not true. You can spend as little as 10 to 20 minutes twice a week and see results. Weight training requires no more time than any other type of exercise.

The American College of Sports Medicine advises a routine of 8 to 10 exercises, each with 8 to 12 repetitions, at least twice a week. We are not talking bench pressing 200 pounds here. Rather, we are talking about picking up a 5-pound weight (more for the guys) and gradually increasing this amount. To follow such a minimal routine with gradual increases will make weight training easy and user friendly—something you can do when you stumble out of bed in the morning or while you're watching your favorite morning show in your bathrobe.

Remember, when you start weight training, you may spend as little as 10 minutes, a couple of times a week, then gradually increase the following variables:

- The amount of weight
- The number of sets (a set is 8 to 12 repetitions)
- The number of different exercises
- The amount of time spent exercising

Remember, the optimal goal with weight training is not to bulk up (unless that is your personal intent) but to maintain your youth and to have a stronger body so that you can lift the 20-pound dog food bag from the truck and carry the dry cleaning at the same time. You will find that within a few weeks, you will start to feel stronger, and in a couple of months, your body will take on a youthful, toned look—not one that is cumbersome or muscle-bound. The added benefit of an increased metabolic rate (more calories burned) will make weight training well worth the effort.

Table 4.1 Weight Training Winners

- Keeps you looking young and toned.
- Increases lean muscle mass and speeds metabolism.
- Protects against bone thinning (osteoporosis).
- Gives you variety in your workout.
- Helps to improve posture.

Red Flag

Before you run out and buy weights or an ab machine, thinking this is the perfect solution to flattening a sagging belly, heed this warning: building abdominal muscles under a layer of fat can make you look even fatter. The idea that you can spot-reduce is nothing but a big myth. When your body loses fat, it loses it from all of the areas where it is stored, not just one, and the exercise that burns fat the quickest is aerobic.

Spice It Up!

Remember when you were a child? You'd eat dinner quickly, then run outside to meet the "gang" for active play. How times have changed! Now most of us eat a heavy meal, then go nest on the couch, waiting for those calorie-laden, cheese stuffed manicotti to appear as new bumps, bulges, and dimples on our thighs or belly.

If you want to look young and feel young, you're now going to have to *think young!* In that regard, it is time to get up, get moving, and have some fun while you do it. You can incorporate creative diversity in your exercise routine by mixing your crunches and your light weights with some type of active or aerobic exercise such as water sports with your children, biking, hiking with a group of friends, or mall walking. Just make sure your active play gets your heart rate up over a sustained amount of time (at least 20 minutes, 3 times a week) so the pounds disappear. Unless you lose body fat, the size and power of those ab muscles from all the crunches are not going to show. And after all, if you work hard to get those amazing muscles, they may as well be admired.

If you are already fit and exercising regularly, you're halfway there toward looking and feeling younger. The second half of the equation is to add some *variation* to your routine such as *spinning* (cycling at high speeds for long periods often done in groups), skating, singles tennis, racquetball, or basketball. Alternating days with various types of exercise and activities will keep your routine diversified. It will also reduce the chances of straining a particular muscle group or joint, not to mention help you to stick with the EAT Plan. Consider weight training 2 days a week and some type of aerobic exercise or activity on another 2 or 3 days.

Whatever you do, make sure your exercise routine is creative, innovative, and anything but *routine!* Exercise and activity have to be fun and fit easily into your lifestyle in order to become a true habit or life-style change. When exercise becomes a part of your daily life, just like brushing and flossing your teeth or moisturizing your face, the chances are greater that you will benefit from it. A revealing study conducted at Harvard Medical School found the strongest predictor for keeping off the weight you lose is to keep exercise a regular part of your daily routine. In contrast, the study revealed that watching television seems to promote weight gain. If you are "tuning in" to the latest sitcom, be sure it is while you're walking on your treadmill or you may be "filling out" more than you anticipated.

> **Just the Facts**
> Don't forget the importance of social support (see page 39)
> and your Circle of Ten as you head out the door to burn those
> 200+ calories. While you can pick up a book or video to learn
> all about exercising, if you joined an aerobics or spinning class,
> or a group of avid walkers, you may just get an extra immune
> boost. Check your local paper or YMCA for information on group
> activities.

Allow for R&R

You don't have to exercise 7 days a week to be fit. In fact, most exercise physiologists say that rest is the other half of a workout. Athletes have learned that peak performance comes from allowing periods of rest between their training sessions. Many coaches and athletes use the terms ''rest'' and ''recovery'' interchangeably, but rest actually refers to doing nothing, while recovery is the period immediately following a workout when your body adjusts to the exercise before it returns to its resting state.

By resting, you allow the body a chance to adjust to the stress put upon it by weight training, running, or other aerobic activities. When you slowly increase the frequency of your workouts, their length or intensity, and then you rest for a certain time, your body becomes stronger and more fit. When you weight-train, even with light weights, it is best to lift 2 or 3 times a week with 24 to 36 hours of rest between sessions. Over time, your goal should be to add days and alternate upper body and lower body routines.

Overtraining increases the likelihood of injury, sickness, and fatigue. While regular, consistent exercise boosts your immune system, excessive exercise (to the point of exhaustion) or overtraining can negatively affect your immune system by pouring adrenaline and cortisol into the bloodstream. These emergency hormones help you cope with the physical stress but can also increase your likelihood of illness. Overexercising can also cause fatigue, insomnia, and lack of interest in sex. If you want to exercise frequently, alternate between light and heavy training days.

Early Bird or Night Owl

What's the best time to exercise? Although you will hear arguments about the best time of day to work out, we think the absolute best time is ... whenever you'll do it. The biggest complaint we hear from seminar participants is the lack of time to exercise. So, what we recommend is a little time management. Using the following questions, figure out when the best time is for you.

Become an Exercise Efficiency Expert

Assess your habits:

- Are you exhausted at night but more energetic in the morning?
- Can you use the treadmill or other equipment while watching your favorite daytime or evening television show?
- Do you talk on the phone all day at work? Would a headset allow you to move around? Or can you deliver that occasional message instead of sending an e-mail to someone else in the building?
- Are you a procrastinator and always save exercise for late in the day—only to be too tired?
- Are you stressed in the late afternoon and need to unwind?
- Is your schedule too full to add another thing in the morning?

Table 4.2 Age Deactivating Benefits of Regular Exercise

- Slows aging
- Keeps you looking young
- Increases energy level
- Reduces stress, anxiety and depression
- Improves sleep
- Improves focus and concentration
- Enhances self-esteem
- Helps maintain normal weight
- Helps with weight loss
- Decreases heart disease and cancer risk
- Increases HDL cholesterol
- Decreases triglycerides
- Lowers blood pressure
- Controls blood sugar levels
- Improves bone density
- Lowers risk of osteoporosis
- Increases fitness needed for better sex
- Boosts immune system

If you procrastinate, then get your exercise done first thing upon arising in the morning. If you are slow to move yet energetic at night, perhaps an after-dinner session is best for you. Get a partner to join in the fun. You can encourage each other, particularly on those days when you'd even dust to get out of exercising!

Keep in mind that you have the greatest chance for success when you are in control of your time and design the plan that works with your life. Check out Table 4.2 for more reasons to keep weight training and moving that body more.

Red Flag

Don't forget to drink lots of water when you exercise. Dehydration reduces blood volume, and the decrease in fluid reaching the brain hinders its efficiency. The result to your body is the feeling of exhaustion. Drinking too little water during your activities negatively affects your speed, endurance, and strength, not to mention that you may feel dizzy, nauseated, or have cramps. Being even slightly dehydrated can reduce your concentration and slow blood circulation. Thirst does not prevent or predict dehydration so it is very important to drink water on a regular schedule instead of waiting until you are thirsty—which sometimes is too late.

Addicted to Exercise?

Unlike Seth, who was addicted to lethargy, there are a host of people who are actually addicted to exercise. When we mention exercise in our seminars, they immediately jump out of their chairs and ask, "When do we start?" We tag these people "fitness fanatics," as they crave the exercise high or work to reinforce their self-esteem. The reason behind the addiction stems from the positive mood boost received from the burst of *endorphins,* the body's natural pain relievers, and other brain chemicals during exercise.

Problems arise when the fitness fanatic's life revolves around her workout to the point of ignoring family and friends, even work, and maybe putting her health at risk. With some addicts, the incredible exercise "high" can be used to escape from a deeper problem. In fact, people with obsessive-compulsive disorder, as well as those with eating disorders, are particularly at risk.

If this description sounds too much like you or someone you know, take the following quiz. Answering "yes" to one or more of the questions may put you at high risk for exercise addiction.

The solution? Seek counseling with a licensed mental health professional. Now that may be one smart move on your part!

Fit or Fanatic?

1. Do you exercise when you are injured or sick?
2. Do you continue to work out even when your doctor has advised you to stop?
3. Have you missed an important personal engagement because you just had to work out?
4. Would you prefer to go for a 10-mile run rather than spend time with family or friends?
5. Do you crave the mood boost you get from exercise?
6. If you miss a workout, do you feel irritable or depressed?
7. Would you jog in inclement weather, such as a thunderstorm or when it's icy cold?
8. Do friends and family members complain about your exercise time?

Play Hard, But Play Safe

If you haven't moved off the sofa in a very long time, are age 45 or above, or have a chronic medical condition, have a checkup before you start weight training or any other type of exercise. You may also want to see a physical therapist to be sure you are exercising correctly, especially if you have a problem with joint pain or mobility. Not only will you not receive full benefit if an exercise is not done correctly, but you may even worsen any pain or ailment. Your doctor can arrange a visit with a physical therapist who is specially trained to teach exercises that achieve the maximum benefit.

Finding the time to exercise may seem more difficult than

actually performing the activity, but once you begin, you will be surprised at how you will come to depend on this time of movement and activity. Your overall attitude toward life will improve, and you may even find yourself hunting for fun activities on your day off because the boost of endorphins makes you feel so good.

No Time for Stress-Aging

Now that you know why stress-aging is a serious malady in America today, we need to talk about your commitment to following the EAT Plan. There can be no more excuses about lack of time to make such life-style changes as moving around more. Consider the alternative. Do you have time for stress-aging and the deleterious health consequences it brings, not to mention the way you look . . . old?

The bottom line is: You now know the secrets behind the Fountain of Youth. As you turn the page and start the EAT Plan, realize that this knowledge is power. Knowing why unhealthy life-style habits can rob you of youthfulness and vitality is important so you can make necessary adjustments.

Starting today, you can do something positive to counteract stress-aging. As you start the six Age Deactivators, not only will you look and feel younger, but you will reap the important benefit of increasing longevity and living stronger all your life.

Part II

Part II

Chapter 5

Stay Young with the Six-Step EAT Plan

After reading about the host of scientific research in the first four chapters, you are beginning to understand why the EAT Plan is your Energy Action Team—and necessary to deactivate stress-aging. Nutritionists know that eating the right foods can help you look and feel young, improve energy, and enhance mental productivity. Now the next six chapters, containing our EAT Plan, will let you in on these secrets!

Your Energy Action Team consists of six Age Deactivators that will liberate you with a revolutionary, nutritional *stay young program,* as you learn to:

1. EAT to stay young and disease-free.
2. EAT to improve mental attitude and performance.
3. EAT to look young.
4. EAT to stay strong and stand tall.
5. EAT to sleep well and feel rested.
6. EAT to balance hormones and feel young.

Each of these Age Deactivators plays an important role in stopping stress-aging. As you read each deactivator, you may see some of the foods or supplements or life-style changes recommended more than once. This is intentional because we address each issue from immunity to looks to sleep to hormones separately. At the end, you will have built a food, supplement, exercise, and relaxation schedule for your individual needs.

We recommend starting with Age Deactivator 1, *Eat Your Weedies*, so you can get the healing effects of foods that are proven to boost your immune system and help control the stress in stress-aging.

Once you've accomplished this first Age Deactivator, progress through Deactivators 2 to 6, until you can say with pride, *"Go ahead. Guess my age!"*

Age Deactivator 1

Eat Your Weedies:

EAT to Stay Young and Disease-Free

Have you made it to the first week of the EAT Plan without
another gray hair? We surely hope so! If you are like most of
our clients, you are anxious to get started and turn back the clock
before Father Time claims any more of your youthful good looks.

In this first Age Deactivator, you will learn to put the brakes
on stress-aging by eating a special grouping of antioxidant
foods—yes, we did say EATING—scientifically proven to fight
disease, boost immune function, and help you look and feel your
best—no matter what your age.

In Chapter 3, you learned all about the immune-boosting benefits of eating these youth-enhancing and healing foods. Now you
will take this knowledge and implement it into your daily routine.
The goal? You will do this for seven days—the first week of the
EAT Plan. Then each subsequent week, as you add another Age
Deactivator to your routine, we will remind you to continue
''Eating Your Weedies.'' Our hope is that eating these foods will
become a natural part of your diet, and not only will you feel
healthier and more energetic (two amazing attributes of youth),

but your body will stand strong against the stressors that come your way.

A Quick and Easy Stress-Aging Cure?

"Great! Now if you'll just tell me where I can buy this stay-young food, I'll be on my way." Julie, a vibrant public relations manager for a computer company, was so enthusiastic that it exhausted us just talking with her. Not only did she want some special "magic" food to keep her young, she wanted it *right now*.

Aren't we all that way? We abuse our bodies and ignore our diet for years, until we come to a point of awakening when we want the "quick and easy stress-aging cure." If only it were that simple! We had to tell Julie that, as nutritionists, we wholeheartedly agree with philosopher H. L. Mencken when he said, "For every complex problem there is a simple solution, and it is wrong."

Of course, that response wasn't what Julie had in mind, and she pressed on, "But I came here to get the plan—the EAT Plan. Isn't this some prepackaged food or drink you can purchase and eat three times a day?" Well, Julie, if there was a guaranteed "Fountain of Youth" we could package and distribute, there would be no need for antiaging seminars or lifesaving tips such as those in this chapter!

Fueling Your Mercedes-Benz

Age Deactivator 1 is based on eating the exact foods to feel healthy, have energy, and stay young. You may be wondering how "eating your weedies" will work to do this. Look at your body as your personal means of transportation—a car, if you will. Now whether you look at your body like a much-desired Mercedes, a reliable sport utility vehicle, or a dented and scratched secondhand pickup truck, it still needs regular care and maintenance to work for you each day. Just like your car needs the proper gasoline and oil to make it run reliably, our bodies need the right balance of protein, carbohydrate, and fat to stay well, as well as a host of vitamins, minerals, antioxidants, phytochemicals, and known and little-known nutrients that help to balance it all.

As you read in Chapter 3, we have come a long way from the Home Economics teacher's advice to eat a variety of food from the "four food groups." Researchers have now discovered in foods some very powerful substances that can actually change the aging process and protect against diseases that occur with age. These are the foods that will be the basis of your Age Deactivator 1.

We have many clients, like Julie, who tell us they don't want to have to think about what to eat, saying, "Just tell me what to do, and I'll do it." At the same time, we have a nation of compulsive dieters who are striving to be thinner at the cost of nutrition and their health. Imagine choosing low-octane gas for a car that needs high octane. You'll pay for the damage—sooner if not later.

No More Quick Fixes

Perhaps one of the greatest motivators in creating the EAT Plan came from a 37-year-old bank executive, Caroline, who was also the single parent of three. We met Caroline at a seminar in Alabama. While she rarely participated during the active group discussions, she quietly handed Susan this note upon leaving:

Dear Susan,

I heard everything you said today and what a reality check! I'm guilty for falling into the worst eating habits. I've starved myself, then binged on junk food. After a week-long fast-food feast, I shifted into the dieting mode, doing the high-protein diet or the prepackaged high-fiber chocolate shakes—brown gooey liquid in a can. Most recently, I tried the low-fat diet and the only thing I lost was my personality! I was cranky, and everyone around me at home and at work knew to stay out of my way.

Yes, I do need help, and I'm willing to do what it takes. As a single mom of three boys, I have no time to plan meals, much less prepare them when I get home. I'm also a bank officer, and I need to look great and feel energetic to compete in this corporate world.

While I envy Oprah's new athletic body, I surely don't have the resources to hire my own fitness consultant or chef to keep me on track. Can't you give me some simple, straightforward solutions to eating that will help me once and for all—eat right to stay young?

Regards,
Caroline

Your Simple, Straightforward Solutions to Stress-Aging

In response to Caroline's request—and the request of hundreds of clients—we have put together some *simple, straightforward solutions* to stopping stress-aging, and the first one is the *Rejuvenating Seven-Day Meal Plan.*

Remember how we discussed the Circle of Ten in Chapter 2? These are ten people or team players who surround us with love and support, and *psychologically* help us deal with the stress of living. When these team players listen to us or offer words of comfort, we feel affirmed and loved. Now, we want you to put together your Circle of Ten foods that can do the same. (No, the foods will *not* listen to you or love you, but you will *love* them!) These Circle of Ten foods will support you *physiologically* and help you deal with the stress of living while preventing stress-aging.

As you incorporate Age Deactivator 1 into your lifestyle, we want you to eat at least five of these foods each day, so be sure to pick foods that you enjoy and that you will eat regularly. Remember that these foods are not the only ones you will eat. They are just the backbone or framework for your deactivating plan to stop stress-aging.

Step 1: Select five foods from this list of potent antioxidant fruits or vegetables:

Apple	Mango
Apricots	Melon
Banana	Onions
Beets	Oranges or orange juice
Bell peppers	Pear
Blackberries	Pineapple
Blueberries	Pink grapefruit
Broccoli	Plums
Brussels sprouts	Raisins
Cabbage	Raspberries
Carrots	Red grapes
Cauliflower	Romaine or other leaf lettuce
Corn	Spinach
Eggplant	Strawberries
Kale, collards, or other greens	Sweet potatoes
Kiwi	Tea
Kohlrabi	Tomatoes or tomato juice

Bright Idea!

Apricots, pineapple, papaya, melon, mango, strawberries, kiwi, banana, raspberries, blueberries, and blackberries all make great additions to plain yogurt, frozen yogurt, or cottage cheese.

Step 2: Select two foods from the following list:

Brown rice	Oatmeal or oat products
Corn	Pasta
Grains that are new or different	Whole grain cereal
(couscous, millet, arborio rice,	Whole grain bread
orzo, or barley)	

Lingo Lowdown

Ever tried *kohlrabi?* It is also called a cabbage turnip and is very high in vitamin C. Kohlrabi can be used as a cabbage, or you can sauté it in vegetable broth, drain, and top with cheddar cheese.

Step 3: Select three foods from the following list:

Beans or peas	Low-fat
Eggs or egg substitute	cheeses
Fish or shellfish	Nuts
Lean meat	Skim milk
	Yogurt

Bright Idea!

To use fat-free or low-fat cheese in a recipe, first shred or grate the cheese. Toss this with a little cornstarch to coat before you try to melt it.

Step 4: Now write down your Circle of Ten foods in the given spaces:

1.   6.

2.   7.

3.   8.

4.   9.

5.   10.

Cathy's Circle of Ten consists of these foods:

1. Spinach or romaine lettuce
2. Tomatoes
3. Orange juice or grapefruit juice
4. Dried fruit
5. Carrots
6. Pasta
7. Cheese
8. Skim milk
9. Whole grain cereal or oatmeal
10. Eggs or egg substitute

Susan's Circle of Ten looks like this:

1. Skim milk
2. Cereal (Cheerios or Shredded Mini-Wheats)
3. Grape juice or orange juice blends (orange-banana)
4. Strawberries
5. Bananas
6. Tuna
7. Whole grain breads
8. Peanut butter or nuts
9. Bell peppers and onions
10. Red leaf lettuce

Although our Circle of Ten foods are different, all of the choices we made are scientifically proven to help keep us disease-free, energetic, and feeling young. See how many of your choices are in the Top Ten list below and consider adding some of these to your list. Research has consistently documented health benefits associated with regular consumption of these foods.

Top Ten Youth Boosters

1. Leafy greens
2. Oatmeal
3. Skim milk
4. Tomatoes, beets
5. Red grapes, strawberries

6. Orange juice
7. Broccoli
8. Nuts or avocado
9. Eggs
10. Fish

Now that you've chosen your Circle of Ten for Week One of the EAT Plan, we want you to THINK TEN throughout your day, and adding the ten immune-boosting foods to your normal menu is one easy way to do it. Here's a sample seven-day menu using Cathy's Week One food choices (Circle of Ten foods are noted with circles).

Cathy's Sample Seven-Day Revitalizing Menu

Day 1

Breakfast
○ Orange juice
○ Whole grain cereal or oatmeal
○ Skim milk
Banana

The Lowdown on Milk and Dairy Products: Low-fat dairy products such as low-fat milk, buttermilk, cheese and cheese products, cottage cheese, ice milk, and yogurt will help protect you from several serious problems associated with aging. Studies show that a diet high in low-fat dairy products and fruits and vegetables significantly lowers blood pressure. The calcium and vitamin D in dairy products helps to keep bones strong and prevent osteoporosis and fractures.

Midmorning
○ Cappuccino with skim milk
Red grapes

The Lowdown on Red Grapes: A superantioxidant called activin has recently been discovered inside the seeds of red grapes. By-products of the red grape, such as wine, juice, or seeds, may offer significant protection against certain types of cancer, heart disease, rheumatoid arthritis, cataracts, and many other chronic and degenerative diseases. Some studies show that activin is up to seven times more powerful as an antioxidant than vitamins C, E, and beta-carotene. This may explain why red wine is more healthful than white wine in protecting you from heart disease. Earlier studies have touted the cancer-fighting properties of resveratrol, a compound extracted from red grape skins. Recent studies conclude that a glass of wine a day may also reduce the risk of age-associated vision loss.

Lunch
○ Vegetable soup (made with crushed tomatoes and chopped onions, carrots, celery, and other favorite vegetables)
○ Greek salad with feta cheese

Red Flag

Don't let lack of time stop you from staying on the EAT Plan. If you don't have time to make vegetable salads for lunch or dinner (or snack for that matter!), choose from the myriad of prepackaged salads available at most supermarkets. You can also find washed baby carrots, chopped broccoli, red and green cabbage, cauliflower and broccoli florets that are ready to eat.

Midafternoon
○ String cheese

Bright Idea!
Keep low-fat or nonfat string cheese in your refrigerator at
work and at home for a high-protein, high-calcium quick snack.

Dinner
○ Pasta with tomato sauce
○ Caesar salad
Italian bread

The Lowdown on Tomatoes: Preliminary research confirms
that the potent antioxidant lycopene, which is prominent in tomatoes, may be more powerful than beta-carotene, alpha-carotene,
and vitamin E. This antioxidant is associated with protection
against heart disease and certain cancers such as prostate and
lung cancer. Cooking tomatoes releases the lycopene and makes
it available for absorption in your body.

Bright Idea!
For easy garlic bread, spray with olive oil Pam and sprinkle
with garlic salt and Italian herbs, then toast under the broiler
until brown.

Day 2

Breakfast
○ Grapefruit juice
○ Whole grain cereal
○ Skim milk
○ Dried fruit

Midmorning
Nonfat yogurt

Lunch
○ Romaine salad with sundried tomatoes, Gorgonzola cheese, and walnuts sprinkled with a dash of flavored olive oil
Whole grain roll

The Lowdown on Olive Oil: Olive oil is a monounsaturated fat that has also been promoted recently as a heart-healthy oil that is preferable to other vegetable oils and margarine. In Mediterranean countries, olive oil is widely used both for cooking and as a salad oil. Breast cancer rates are 50 percent lower in Mediterranean countries than in the United States.

Midafternoon
Peanut butter crackers

Dinner
Baked chicken
Brown rice
○ Steamed carrots and fresh broccoli florets
○ Sliced tomatoes

The Lowdown on Broccoli: This green tree-like vegetable is full of indoles, isothiocyanates, and sulforaphane—phytochemicals that have been shown to trigger enzyme systems that block or suppress cellular DNA damage. In other words, it packs an amazing power punch of healing nutrition! If you really want the highest concentration of these cancer-fighting compounds, get broccoli sprouts at your local health food store. The sprouts have 10 to 100 times more sulphoraphane than mature broccoli.

Day 3

Breakfast
○ Orange juice
○ Whole grain cereal
○ Skim milk
Strawberries

Midmorning
○ String cheese

Lunch
○ Grilled veggie sub sandwich
○ Raw baby carrots

Bright Idea!

To make roasted veggies, preheat the oven to 350°. Thinly slice yellow and zucchini squash, mushrooms, eggplant, and onions. Add chunks of red and green pepper, asparagus, and any other favorite vegetables. Place these veggies on a baking sheet being careful not to overlap any. Spray with olive oil Pam, then sprinkle with favorite spices (onion or garlic powder, rosemary, basil, oregano). Bake at 350° for 30 minutes, turning after 15 minutes. Stuff veggies inside a whole wheat sub roll, and sprinkle with feta cheese, if desired. Also good with balsamic vinegar sprinkled on top.

Midafternoon
Trail mix

Dinner
Grilled fish
Baked potato (or sweet potato) with nonfat sour cream and
freshly cut chives

○ Broccoli with lemon and Parmesan cheese
○ Raw baby carrots

The Lowdown on Fish: New studies show that eating fish at least once per week can cut the risk of sudden cardiac death. One eleven-year study of 20,551 male physicians found that men who ate fish once a week had half the risk of sudden cardiac death as those who ate fish less than once a month. While this study focused on men, it wouldn't hurt women to get on the bandwagon! Substances in fish called omega-3 fatty acids may have a protective effect against sudden cardiac death, possibly by preventing potentially dangerous arrhythmias or irregular heartbeats. Some heart-healthy fish include:

Anchovies	Sardines
Bluefish	Scallops
Lobster	Tuna
Mackerel	Whitefish
Salmon	

Day 4

Breakfast
○ Piña colada smoothie
Bran muffin

Bright Idea!
Here's how to make a Piña Colada Smoothie: Combine ¼ cup orange juice, ¼ cup piña colada mix (nonalcoholic), ½ cup pineapple juice, 1 cup nonfat vanilla yogurt, and 3 ice cubes. Blend until creamy and smooth.

Midmorning
○ Hard-boiled egg

Lunch
Sliced turkey
Barbequed beans
○ Cole slaw (add finely chopped carrots and tomatoes)

Midafternoon
○ Peanuts

Dinner
○ Risotto with veggies (carrots, broccoli, onions, or other favorites)
○ Romaine salad sprinkled with fresh shredded Parmesan cheese
Green tea

The Lowdown on Green Tea: Green tea is a powerful antioxidant and may help in preventing liver, pancreatic, breast, lung, esophageal, and skin cancers. It has also been found to aid in reducing the risk of cardiovascular disease and stroke, and some new studies indicate that it may help in preventing osteoporosis. Researchers report that a nontoxic chemical found in green tea, *epigallocatechin-3 gallate,* acts against *urokinase* (an enzyme crucial for cancer growth). One cup of green tea contains between 100 and 200 milligrams of this antitumor ingredient.

Day 5

Breakfast
○ Orange juice
○ Whole grain cereal
○ Skim milk
Banana

Midmorning
One-half peanut butter and jelly sandwich

Lunch
○ Veggie omelet sprinkled with shredded cheddar cheese (top with tomato salsa, if you like)
○ Spinach salad

The Lowdown on Spinach: *You've probably heard a lot about homocysteine* lately on the news. This naturally occurring blood protein promotes artery clogging, and is a by-product of meals high in protein. With the latest health concerns about *homocysteine,* nutritionists tell us the cure is simple: add more folic acid. Folic acid dramatically lowers elevated levels of homocysteine in the blood. The risk of age-related macular degeneration (AMD), the leading cause of blindness in older people, is also significantly decreased by eating this green vegetable. Spinach is high in folic acid, a nutrient crucial during early pregnancy to prevent neural-tube defects in children, and this power vegetable is also abundant in beta-carotene, vitamins A and C, and potassium.

You can easily get the minimum daily intake of folic acid (400 micrograms) by adding the following to your diet:

Dark green vegetables
Fruits, especially citrus fruits or juices
Whole grains
Enriched breakfast cereals

Midafternoon
○ Trail mix

Dinner
○ Pasta with tomato and meat sauce (use freshly ground turkey breast or a mixture of ground turkey or chicken and lean

ground beef. Another excellent beef substitute is the new all-vegetable protein crumbles, a soy protein beef substitute available in your frozen foods section.
○ Caesar salad
Garlic bread

Day 6

Breakfast
○ Grapefruit juice
Bran muffin
○ Cappuccino with skim milk

Midmorning
○ String cheese

Lunch
○ Mozzarella cheese and tomato sandwich (can also be toasted)

Bright Idea!
Blend the following herbs in equal parts and store in an airtight container: rosemary, black pepper, red pepper, onion powder, garlic powder, basil, oregano, and lite salt. Shake herbs before using, and put 1 teaspoon of mixture on a plate. Pour 1 to 2 tablespoons olive oil over this, and use to spread on sandwiches or as a dipping oil for breads.

Midafternoon
Nonfat yogurt

Dinner
Filet mignon with garlic cloves
○ Baked potato with shredded sharp cheese on top
○ Spinach salad

The Lowdown on Garlic: Garlic contains chemicals that act like ACE (angiotensin-converting enzyme) inhibitors, prescription drugs that are commonly given to lower blood pressure and protect the heart. Supplements of garlic reduce blood pressure by dilating blood vessels. In fact, some studies have revealed that ingesting one or two cloves of fresh garlic daily can lower mildly elevated blood pressure an average of 8 percent in 1 to 3 months. Further research has found that garlic and onions can block formation of nitrosamines, powerful carcinogens that target several sites in the body, usually the liver, colon, and breasts. The more pungent the garlic or onion, the more abundant the chemically active sulfur compounds that provide the protection.

Day 7

Breakfast
○ Orange juice
○ Egg and cheese on wheat toast

Midmorning
Biscotti
○ Skim milk

Lunch
○ Tuna salad served on romaine lettuce (add diced apple or finely chopped carrots to tuna salad for texture and new flavor)
○ Tomato slices
Fresh fruit

Midafternoon
○ Trail mix

Dinner
Chicken stir-fry
Brown rice

○ Steamed baby carrots
○ Romaine salad

Now, based on your own Circle of Ten, plug these foods into your daily meals or menus to improve your defense against stress-aging. If you find yourself getting tired of eating a particular food, remember that there are many more with disease-fighting properties listed here or in Chapter 3. Just pick a new one and include it in your circle. Our clients tell us they post their Circle of Ten on the refrigerator as a constant reminder during meal time to add healing foods.

Your Circle of Ten will become your personalized rejuvenating meal plan to keep stress-aging at bay. Yes, we told you this would be a *simple, straightforward solution* to stopping stress-aging! Now do you believe us? Keep reading for more age deactivating tips.

Immune Booster or Immune Buster?

We all have days when the stress just keeps hitting. One mother of teenagers said she felt like life was a nonstop treadmill. "I keep trying to find the off button, but can't. I'd even like to slow down for a day or two, but the stressors keep zapping me."

When you are faced with high stress and need some additional comfort, don't head for the Little Debbie cakes. Instead, try some of these Immune Booster foods instead of the usual Immune Buster high-fat or high-calorie foods.

Immune Busters	Immune Booster
Bacon, egg, and cheese biscuit	Veggie omelet
Burger	Veggie sub with cheese
French fries	Side salad with a lot of cut-up veggies
Soft drinks	Fruit or juice
Potato chips	Dried fruit or trail mix
Ice cream	Fruit sorbet
Onion dip	Bean dip
Hot dog	Peanut butter sandwich
Pepperoni and sausage pizza	Veggie pizza

Bright Idea!
Make scrumptious baked French fries. Preheat oven to 350°. Cut a potato into 3-inch slices lengthwise, and place on a baking sheet. Spray potatoes with olive oil Pam, then sprinkle with your favorite herbs, salt, and pepper. Bake for 30 minutes, turning frequently.

Sometimes the original food does not need a total substitute but just an additional immune-boosting food to make it beneficial. For example, if you like barbeque chicken, add baked beans and cole slaw to your meal to get some immune-boosting phytochemicals. If you like steak, go for the smallest and leanest cut like filet mignon, then add a steaming baked potato topped with shredded low-fat cheddar cheese and a tossed romaine salad or a bowl of roasted seasonal vegetables (see recipe on page 110 to boost your dinner's phytochemical content.

Just the Facts
If you are a strict vegetarian eating no dairy foods, choose calcium-rich foods such as legumes, calcium-fortified juices, soy nuts, calcium-fortified soy milk, and molasses to help meet your calcium needs. Also make sure to eat artichokes, broccoli, Brussels sprouts, cabbage, carrots, celery, lima beans, snap beans, spinach, and Swiss chard.

It's Back to Basics Again: Count Those Calories

Interestingly, since most everyone you know is on a diet at least some of the time, the number of obese people in America is swelling—literally. The good news is that certain foods can increase your good health and lifespan, yet there is some bad news, too. According to a Louis Harris and Associates survey in 1997, Americans are fatter than ever before. Seventy-four percent of Americans 25 or older are overweight, up from 71 percent in 1996, 69 percent in 1994, 66 percent in 1992, and only 59 percent 10 years ago.

"Come on. It's just fifteen pounds. Quit being so picky!" Tom, a 49-year-old attorney didn't believe us when we said that taking off 5 or 10 pounds would help reduce his elevated blood pressure. Still, when his doctor gave him the choice between losing weight or taking two different blood pressure medications, Tom began to take this slight weight increase to heart—literally!

Weighing as little as 10 or 15 pounds over your desired weight can exacerbate a heart condition, elevate blood pressure and cholesterol, and even increase your risk of age-related diabetes and certain cancers, not to mention make you look and feel older than you are.

But there is hope! According to Harvard researchers, while gaining weight can increase the chance of ailments such as hypertension, losing weight will reduce that risk. These findings were from the Nurses' Health Study, an ongoing study of 82,473 United States female nurses started in 1976, and reported in the *Annals of Internal Medicine* (1998).

"Okay. I know this spare tire is going to cause me trouble someday, and my blood pressure is borderline high. Yet I swear I diet religiously." Patsy patted her expanding girth and told us about a recent semistarvation grapefruit and steak diet, on which she lost 9 pounds in 2 weeks, then gained them all back as soon as she began eating normally again. Patsy pleaded for answers to her ever-growing concern with obesity.

Stop the Dieting Merry-Go-Round

When will America wake up? Is it any coincidence that the more we diet, the more stress we create in our lives, and the fatter we get? The fatter we get, the more stress we feel, and we go on another diet. It becomes a vicious never-ending cycle of deprivation and failure.

**Weight gain → Diet → Deprivation → Stress →
Binge eating → Weight gain**

Which of the Fad Diets Have You Tried?

- Eating cabbage soup for 7 days
- Skipping a meal a day to reduce calorie intake
- Drinking quarts of ice water to help boost metabolism
- Substituting low-calorie, high-fiber shakes for real food
- Drastically restricting whole groups of food like fat or carbohydrates
- Eating grapefruit before meals to burn more fat
- Eating virtually no fat to lose fat
- Using pills or supplements designed to boost metabolism

When you look at this list of popular weight loss methods, it becomes apparent that most people today are not starving for food. Rather the real hunger is for surefire ways to get in control of weight problems and return to a normal weight. Keep reading to learn how you can do just that.

For the past decade, the media has misled Americans into thinking that "calories no longer count." You've read the headlines:

Eat More, Weigh Less
Count Fats, Not Calories
Calories Don't Count!

Don't believe any of this hype! It is simply not true and could cause you to gain more than years as you age. When it comes to your weight, *calories do count,* and one of the biggest ways that additional calories may show up on your plate is in the portion size.

Until now, we have focused entirely on specific foods you must eat to stay young. Well, now we want you to look at how much you actually eat compared to how much you should eat to stay at a normal weight.

Just the Facts

One of the truths of aging is that, after age 20, your metabolism (or the amount of calories your body burns at rest) slows down an average of 10 percent every decade. If you keep eating at the same rate with the same level of exercise, watch out! Here comes middle-age spread. Yet it doesn't have to be this way. You can stay metabolically active, and Age Deactivator 4 (pages 179 to 199) will teach you how.

When Bigger Is *Not* Better

The fast-food trend of "bigger is better" is certainly capturing a large audience—in more ways than one! The most recent new burger advertised is one-half pound of meat with double cheese and eight slices of bacon. It doesn't take a licensed nutritionist to know that this whopping 1,500 calories and 140 grams of fat is not good for you. Better make sure your affairs are in order if you keep eating like this!

So, you buy the small hamburger to save calories yet still insist on the fries? May want to rethink this one, too. At the American Dietetic Association meeting in 1997, Dr. Lawrence T. P. Stifler, President of Health Management Resources in Boston, reported that the small-size French fries sold today in fast-food restaurants are larger than the large-size French fries were ten years ago. If you think it's amazing that for just a few pennies, you can "supersize" your meals, just remember that you may also be supersizing your body as well.

Let Us Read Your Palm

"You've given us all these wonderful choices of food for our Circle of Ten—pasta, muffins, even filet mignon. Do we eat until we're full? That sounds too good to be true." Well . . . if something sounds too good to be true, it usually is! Seriously, if you ate until you were full—of any food—you'd wear it on your hips or waist for months to come. But you have a built-in portion guide that will help you decide how much is enough—to fill your tummy, satisfy your hunger cravings, and keep your weight at a normal level. The guide? It's your hand.

Look at the palm of your hand to calculate a correct portion. Meals should include three to four servings of food the size of the palm of your hand. If your meal could fit in a bucket better than in your hand, you may need to eat less at each meal or exercise a whole lot more! Remember the data on page 64, suggesting that in animals, eating less led to longer lives. This is an easy way to cut back on unnecessary calories and still enjoy our food.

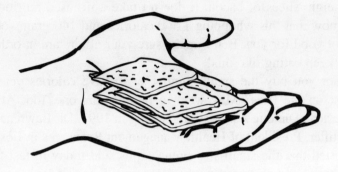

Age Deactivator #1

Personally Speaking

Portion size was brought home to Cathy when she saw an exhibition at the Cummer Museum of Art in Jacksonville, Florida, of porcelain dishes from ancient China. Her husband, Leo, took one look at the miniature plates, and said, "Those must be the snack-size dishes!" Perhaps they were, at least when compared to the oversized dishes most of us use at home. Is it any wonder we are all eating more and wearing the extra calories on our hips, thighs, and waistlines?

Liquid Calories Don't Count . . . Do They?

Another easy way to change the content of your diet and add those necessary phytochemicals so important for deactivating stress-aging is to look at what you drink. The biggest change in the American diet in the nineties so far is the increase in carbonated soft drinks. In fact, carbonated soft drinks are the fastest-growing food/beverage category served at home and in restaurants, according to the NPD Group's Twelfth Annual Report on Eating Patterns in America published in March 1998. Studies show that in 1990, the average American consumed soft drinks on 83 different occasions during the year. In 1997, the number was up to 102 servings a year. This increase is four times that of any other food or beverage item. Also in this category, what once was considered a large drink is now a regular or even a small size. (Other increases in at-home consumption included presweetened cereal, bagels, toaster pastries, and pizza. In restaurants, top increases included French fries, Mexican food, and burgers.)

Although there are beverages on the list of age-deactivating foods, this survey did not find them to be top choices. How about fruit juices, tea, or water to quench that thirst? Remember that what you drink can also be counted in your Circle of Ten and help you get those age deactivators in for the day.

Designer Supplements

Creating your Circle of Ten foods is a big step in stopping stress-aging. Nonetheless, research shows that people under stress tend to eat less well than those who are not stressed. If you find that you eat less or eat more under stress, examine what you are eating. None of our clients have ever noted an improvement in nutrition when stressed! Take Kristin, for example. This first-year medical student goes to school full-time and also works 20 hours a week to help make ends meet. Her life dream of becoming a heart surgeon is admirable, but Kristin's eating habits are anything but.

"I usually have a yogurt and Coke before classes, then grab some peanuts midafternoon with another Coke. When I get to the nursing home where I work, I try to grab some cheese crackers and coffee out of a vending machine. I get home late and I'm too tired to cook, so I settle for a piece of fruit and some ice cream."

Kristin lost weight doing this "hit and miss" eating, but it quickly showed in her face and health. By the end of the first semester of med school, she had bronchitis and was on her second set of antibiotics.

As we shared with Kristin, by eating from your Circle of Ten, day in and day out, you will fortify your stress-aging defenses and be stronger for the long run. Yet for those times when eating well is overshadowed by stress, as Kristin experienced trying to go to school and work, there are some backup systems to get you through. One of these is the use of supplements.

When it comes to supplement use, we believe you can design your own plan using the available supplements on the market. As nutritionists, we find it frustrating that we can't always find the exact mix or blend of supplements we want based on the current need. Whether from illness or increased stress, our bodies change but the bottled supplements seem to stay the same.

You can pick and choose from the available supplements at your local pharmacy or grocery store to make your own Designer Supplement Plan until the manufacturers catch up with the ground-breaking research. Here's a start on what you might choose:

1. Vitamin C: 250–1,000 mg daily especially during times of stress or when fruit and vegetable intake is low.
2. Vitamin E: 200–400 IU daily.
3. Multivitamin/mineral: 100% of the RDA for most vitamins and minerals daily especially during times of stress. Make sure it contains at least 400 IU of folic acid and choose one with a low iron level unless anemic.
4. Calcium supplement: 1,000–1,500 mg daily.
5. Echinacea, as needed for cold defense (read label for dosage).
6. Garlic: Take daily for reducing cardiovascular disease risk.

Hope or Hype?

With all the supplements advertised daily, how do you know what is true and what is hype? We've put together our *Circle of Ten Supplement Guidelines* to help you evaluate new products for safety and effectiveness.

1. Is it a cure-all? If it purports to fix everything from A to Z, well, there's no such thing.
2. Is the majority of support for its use from individuals who feel better or claim it worked for them? These are called *individual testimonials,* and if that's the main basis for the supplement's use, watch out. There's no way to evaluate these personal opinions scientifically, and they have little validity.
3. Is it being promoted on the idea that foods, especially fruits and vegetables, are not nutritionally as good as they once were because our soil is depleted of nutrients? The truth is that plant foods will not grow if the soil is nutrient-deficient. We can maximize the nutrients that are there with our preparation techniques, such as cooking in a small amount of water for a short period of time or eating less-processed plant foods, but they start out nutritionally sound.
4. Is the product sold through a pyramid marketing plan?
5. Is the product recommended as necessary or important for everyone without regard to age, health, diet, or risk?
6. Does the product promise more than seems probable to achieve? Is it too good to be true?
7. Does the cost seem unreasonable?
8. Is the product promoted as a new cure that is being held back by the medical establishment?
9. Are there fewer than three studies from peer-reviewed

scientific journals that support the claims being made about the product?

10. Does the person recommending the product have a financial incentive?

If you answered yes to any of these questions, do some more exploration. It doesn't necessarily mean the product is bad or harmful, but there may not be enough evidence to know. Ask a licensed nutritionist or dietitian for a professional recommendation regarding use of the product. Check with your pharmacist or doctor for another professional opinion. By using our Circle of Ten Guidelines, you can surround yourself with all the information you need to make an informed choice.

One Down, Five to Go

Go ahead and choose your foods and start your Revitalizing Meal Plan today. Try to incorporate the other suggestions such as watching that portion size and supplementing your diet with vitamins and minerals, if you are not eating properly.

Now moving on to Age Deactivator 2, we'll teach you how to eat for comfort and enjoyment, while using that psychological Circle of Ten to heal your mind, body, and soul.

Be Your Own Bodyguard:

EAT to Improve Mental Attitude and Performance

In Chapter 2, you learned about the benefits of soul food to staying young. We discussed the importance of getting in touch with the inner you, the significance of optimism, the dangers of cynicism and pessimism, and how social support can strengthen immunity and improve the quality of your life.

Now we're going to take all the information shared on pages 25 to 46 and help you put these research realities into practice. No one can stop the guaranteed increase in years as we get older. Yet we know you will look and feel younger as you learn to EAT to improve your attitude and mental performance.

Mood Check

Before we dive into the steps for Deactivator 2, let's share a story about one client, Ellen, who wanted help with mood swings. This 34-year-old mother and landscape architect was usually a good-natured person. Even with the normal hormonal changes women experience each month, Ellen had no problem handling small upheavals in mood.

"It's when work stress and family stress hit head-on, usually at the same time, and I feel angry, depressed, and hostile. Sometimes I can balance the stress with getting better sleep or more exercise. But sometimes I just eat . . . and eat and eat and eat. A few weeks ago when I was in charge of giving the new client presentation, I ate nonstop for four days straight without a break, and I'm not talking rabbit food either."

Of course, we thought Ellen was exaggerating a bit. Yet when she showed us her stress-eating marathon menu, we knew she had some hurdles to jump:

Ellen's Marathon Stress-Eating Binge

Day 1

Breakfast:	Waffles with butter and syrup (*real* syrup and *real* butter!)
	Chocolate milk
Midmorning:	Doughnuts at the office (preferably glazed, fried and not just one!)
	Coffee with cream and sugar
Lunch:	Snickers' bar (large size)
	Coke
	One apple
Midafternoon:	A bite or two of whatever anyone is eating that is sweet!
	Jelly beans (the whole bag)
	Coke
Dinner:	Hamburger with lettuce (gee, a green vegetable?)
	Chocolate milkshake (large size)
	Ben and Jerry's Chubby Hubby Ice Cream (1 pint)
Bedtime snack:	Warm, homemade cookies
	Ice cold milk

Lucky for Ellen

Ellen needs to thank her lucky stars that she is a naturally slim person, or she would be wearing all this sugar and fat on each hip with a few inches added to her waistline for good measure! While some talk about working out to have rock-hard abs like a "six-pack," Ellen was working on an entire case!

Does your mood affect the way you eat, as Ellen claims, or do your food choices affect your mood? Quite honestly, for most people, it's some of each. Nonetheless, we want to help you use this food-mood connection to your optimal stay-young benefit as you *eat to improve mental attitude and performance.* The EAT Plan—your Energy Action Team—is designed to help you understand that in the midst of the hustle and bustle of your harried life, you are actually in charge of the way you look and feel. Let's get started!

Step 1: Become the Master of Your Appetite

In our previous book, *I'd Kill for a Cookie* (Dutton, 1997), we talk about the ground-breaking research that showed that women tend to eat more when alone, sad, or stressed while men tend to eat more when they are happy or in a group. Not only did the moods vary by gender, but so did the food choices. Women tended to eat what we call sugar-fat food combinations like desserts (notice Ellen's choices), while men tended to reach more for protein-fat foods like pizza, cheese, nuts, or burgers. What is the common denominator? You guessed it! It's *fat.*

"But *why* do I reach for high-fat foods when stressed, when I know better?" Ellen really wanted to break her love affair with sugar-fat foods before genetics stopped protecting her (around mid-thirties) and she began to look like the sugar-fat addict she was. As we shared with Ellen, the reason we reach for high-fat foods may be in the soothing comfort they give. Basically, foods high in fat make us feel fuller and provide satiety, the feeling of satisfaction when we're finished eating. You may connect some high-fat foods to home, family, or situations that made you feel loved and cared for. Check out the list of Common Comfort Foods, and see which are your favorites during periods of high stress:

Common Comfort Foods

Chicken soup
Cookies
Chocolate
Ice cream
Ginger ale
Mashed potatoes with gravy
Pudding
Macaroni and cheese
Regional or cultural carbohydrate foods such as grits, rye
    bread, spaetzle, pasta, rice, wild rice, oatmeal, or cream of
    wheat

If you are like Ellen and continually look to food to boost your mood when stress hits, you may actually be *activating* stress-aging rather than *deactivating* it. Now that's a problem if you are working to look and feel young again.

Make Comfort Foods Guilt-Free

Even when you feel compelled to eat your favorite comfort food, you are still the Captain of your Ship, or rather, the Master of Your Appetite. You are totally in control of the *amount* you eat. In other words, you can stop after a reasonable portion—enough to satisfy your craving—and then move on with your life. This is what can make your comfort food guilt-free.

So take another look through the list of Common Comfort Foods again on page 130, keeping in mind this time that portion size is important—and for some Common Comfort Foods, we're not talking about what will fit in the palm of your hand! Rather, if chocolate is a comfort for you and helps you to feel loved and even a bit young again, a small candy bar or a few chocolate kisses may do the trick. For peanut lovers, a thick homemade peanut butter cookie with a glass of fat-free milk may quench your craving. Or a small serving of homemade mashed potatoes may help you make it through a rough day if that brings comfort to your body and soul.

"How can just a little bit of comfort food satisfy me? What if I continue to eat and eat, like I used to?" Ellen really wanted to become the Master of her Appetite. We will tell you what we shared with her, that is:

Tip 1: Determine the amount of food you usually eat, e.g. three cookies, or one cup of macaroni and cheese.

Tip 2: Serve yourself one-third to one-half of that amount, e.g. one cookie, or one-half cup of macaroni and cheese.

Tip 3: When you have eaten that portion, stop and ask, *Am I satisfied and in control?*

Remember, comfort food is just that—food. It can temporarily soothe the emotional or psychological part of us that needs some help but the effects are very short-term. This explains why emotional eaters are not satisfied with a small amount; they keep searching for the help they need. Food is merely a distracter, making them feel better only in the short term. If you eat food for comfort daily or several times a week, look for support in other places. Expand your Circle of Ten and deepen those relationships to give you the support you need.

Red Flag

If you can't stop eating or feel that you are out of control, then it's important to know that food is not the issue or the answer. Seek help from a licensed mental health professional to help gain control of your eating (and overeating).

Step 2: Eat Winning Foods to Increase Concentration and Alertness

In addition to the link comfort foods have to your moods, foods that contain protein have been linked with improved concentration and alertness. Likewise, foods that are primarily carbohydrate seem to have a calming effect on our moods. We eat the brownie and actually feel better—for a little while. We feel calmer, less anxious, and relaxed, but the effect lasts only for an hour or two. Because we do feel temporarily better, the next time we feel stressed, we reach for carbohydrate foods again.

On the other hand, a food containing protein will give a temporary boost in alertness and concentration, allowing you to focus on the task at hand. Protein is also satisfying, so it should curb hunger longer than carbohydrate foods eaten alone and provide a feeling of satisfaction or fullness.

To improve concentration and alertness, don't skip meals, spread your calories out throughout the day, and choose from our *Gold Medal List of Winning Foods* when you need a boost in concentration and alertness.

Gold Medal List of Winning Foods for Concentration and Alertness

1. Skim milk
2. Yogurt
3. Low-fat cheese
6. Shellfish
7. Egg or egg substitute
8. Beans and peas

| 4. Turkey or chicken breast | 9. Soy milk |
| 5. Fish | 10. Peanut butter or nuts |

Of All the Things I've Lost with Time . . . I Miss My Mind the Most

Who hasn't forgotten a date or where they put the checkbook? If memory glitches are bothering you, try these easy ways to reclaim some of that youthful, quick memory:

1. Carry a pad and pencil with you, and write things down. Keep your notes in a place you will see often.
2. Try to pay close attention when people speak or when you read. If you really focus, you will have a better chance of remembering.
3. If you can't remember names, try to link the person's name with a characteristic or behavior that describes the person, such as ''Hyper Harry'' or ''Beautiful Bess.''
4. Organize lists into meaningful categories. If you forget the list, the categories can remind you of items that were there. For example, a grocery list divided into dairy, fruits, frozen foods, meats, cereals, grains, and desserts will help you remember which foods you need when you get to those aisles.
5. Create a mental picture of the thing you need to remember. Concentrate on a color or something unique to trigger your memory later.
6. Eliminate distractions as much as possible. If you make your list with the television on, you may forget something important.
7. Try to keep your office or home organized in a logical way. When things are always kept in the same place, it is easier to remember where they are.

Step 3: Add Foods High in B-Vitamins to Quit Singing the Blues

In addition to comfort foods and carbohydrate or protein foods aiding in mood management, the B-vitamins have been implicated in mood as well. It has long been known that people with B-vitamin deficiencies had mental symptoms like depression, anxiety, and mood swings. Now according to the latest comprehensive studies, folic acid is the one B vitamin that seems to be in the forefront of mood management. A third of the people who suffer from depression have been found to have lower levels of folic acid in the blood. Folic acid is found in green leafy vegetables, beans, peas, peanuts and other legumes, and citrus fruits.

In new research carried out jointly by researchers at Massachusetts General Hospital in Boston and the Baylor Research Institute in Dallas, patients with low folic acid levels were more likely to have melancholia, a type of depression characterized by sadness and declines in mental and physical activity. The 8-week study of 213 patients also found that those with low levels of folic acid were significantly less likely to respond to treatment for depression with fluoxetine (Prozac), a common antidepressant medication.

What does this say to those who are busy "singing the blues"? Better start eating more weedies, especially those green ones! Select from the following foods that pack a folic acid punch.

Folic Acid Mood Elevators

Brewer's yeast	Broccoli
Spinach	Beets
Asparagus	Sunflower seeds
Turnip greens	Kidney beans
Lima beans	Dandelion greens
Beef liver	Cantaloupe
Black-eyed peas	Bean sprouts

Pinto beans   Wheat germ
Parsley   Tofu
Navy beans   Grapefruit juice

Just the Facts

Most multivitamins contain 400 IU of folic acid, and supplements are available alone or in conjunction with other B-vitamins. With the discovery that folic acid reduces the risk of neural tube defects during pregnancy and cardiovascular disease, supplements are much more widely used than before. Note: If you are already eating enough folic acid-rich foods, taking more will not result in improved mood.

Step 4: Use Good Scents to Deactivate Stress-Aging

If you've ever salivated when an aromatic whiff of Mom's homemade chocolate chip cookies drifted your way, or felt alert even before you took that first sip of brewed Java in the morning, then you have successfully used *good scents* or *aromatherapy.*

Lingo Lowdown

- *Aromatherapy* is a type of "nose-mind" therapy that uses fragrances or essential and absolute oils and other substances for physical and psychological benefits.
- *Essential oil* is an extract or essence that's been distilled, usually by steam, from the seed, leaves, stem, flower, bark, root, or other parts of a plant.
- *Absolute oil* is a very concentrated liquid extracted from a plant by alcohol.
- Essential oils are often diluted in a *carrier oil* such as sweet almond, grapeseed, olive, or canola oil before using with massage.

Each of the different aromas or oils has a specific benefit, whether to reduce stress, fight infection, increase productivity, or serve as an aphrodisiac. For example, lavender and spiced apples are said to increase the alpha wave activity in the back of the brain, which leads to relaxation; jasmine or lemon are used to increase beta activity in the front of the brain and heighten alertness.

Although you have probably experienced how odors you like can brighten your positive mood, exactly how aromatherapy works remains a mystery. Researchers do know that when you inhale aromatic molecules, they bind receptors and build electrical impulses that move up the olfactory nerves to the brain. The ultimate target is the limbic system, where your emotions and memory are processed.

Relaxers

Lavender
Chamomile
Sandalwood
Orange blossom
Spiced apples
Vanilla

Invigorators

Spearmint
Pine
Eucalyptus
Jasmine
Lemon or orange

Romance Inducers

Jasmine
Rose
Cinnamon

How to Use Essential Oils

- Inhale the oil by adding 5 to 10 drops to steaming water or to a humidifer.
- Mix 1 teaspoon oil with 1 pint carrier oil, and use as a massage oil.
- Add 5 to 10 drops to warm bath water.
- Mix 5 drops with 1 cup warm water and mist into the air.
- Put 1 to 2 drops on top of a candle's melted wax, and inhale the warm scent.

Step 5: Nurture Your Circle of Ten

Remember the Circle of Ten teammates you defined on page 39? We want you to use these same names and begin to nurture these friendships. Just as you nurture your body to deactivate stress-aging, you must nurture close relationships to get that all-powerful immunity boost.

Follow our ten tips for maintaining stronger, lasting friendships:

Tip 1: Turn *off* the television, and turn *on* to friends. One-on-one contact strengthens friendships and builds memories. If you rarely see each other, communicate frequently by phone or e-mail. Keep the connection alive by sharing your current experiences. Interestingly, a survey of 10,000 Americans by sociologists Geoffrey Godbey at Pennsylvania State University and John Robinson at the University of Maryland found that adults who watch the most television (16 hours a week was average) are the least likely to socialize with friends, take classes, or play sports.

Tip 2: Remember to be appreciative. Everyone needs to feel wanted and important in life. Find ways to thank a friend for a kind word or act, and tell her what it meant to you.

Tip 3: Listen, and really hear what your friend is saying. Everyone counts on friends to be sounding boards when things go well or go poorly. So, make sure you're there when your friend needs to talk.

Tip 4: Enjoy laughter together. Enjoy your friends by making time to laugh, sharing jokes or going to funny movies together.

Tip 5: Support your friend in family relationships. Never criticize the husband, wife, or children of a friend. This behavior divides loyalties and places your friend in a tough bind, having to choose between your friendship and her family.

Tip 6: Show your friends that you think of them even when you're not with them. Sending cards or funny gifts to let them know you remembered them strengthens your bond. For example, if you know they like a certain fragrance, buy a candle with that scent, or bring home a souvenir from a trip that has special meaning for both of you.

Tip 7: Don't keep score. If a disagreement occurs, let it go. Waiting for a friend to apologize or counting who calls who first detracts from the relationship. As friends, we know the other's faults and idiosyncrasies. Being friends means giving acceptance and support—no matter how much you may have argued a week ago.

Tip 8: Be there when times are tough. Even if you don't live in the same town, just a card, a message, or the delivery of food or flowers can remind your friend that you are there in spirit. Often, it's not what you say or the things you give but rather the unspoken message that you are "there through the good times or bad" that supports the relationship.

Tip 9: Be tactfully honest. Friends ask for your opinion because they value it. Because you value your friends, speak the truth using tactfulness. This means telling the truth in a way that is helpful, not hurtful or destructive. In this regard, sometimes the best thing to say is nothing at all!

Tip 10: Enjoy each other. Strong connections help both of you. Enjoy your differences, and celebrate your similarities.

What Type of Support Do You Have?

Now, go back to page 39, and consider your Circle of Ten teammates again. Ask yourself what type of support you can count on from each person. Not everyone in your circle will give you all kinds of support. Emotional support is probably the most important, but you may start a relationship on another level and move up to a different level in the process.

- **Emotional support.** Someone you trust with your most intimate thoughts.
- **Social support.** Someone you enjoy being with to share life experiences.
- **Informational support.** Someone you can ask for advice on major decisions. Many people in professional life look at these individuals as mentors.
- **Practical support.** Someone who will help you out in a pinch. Sometimes, neighbors or coworkers are in this category.

While you are going over each of the four types of support needed to deactivate stress-aging, remember that all these supports are desirable. Using the following space, write down the names of your Circle of Ten supporters. Next to each person's name, write the type of support you get from that person (emotional, social, informational, or practical).

Your Circle of Ten	*Type of Support Provided*
1.	
2.	
3.	
4.	
5.	
6.	
7.	
8.	
9.	
10.	

If your Circle of Ten teammates provide the *emotional and social support* you need, that's great! That's why you chose these ten special people and why you work to have a Circle of Ten supporters. Still, you can also add a new Circle of Ten supporters to cover the practical and informational support that is necessary to deactivate stress-aging. This Circle of Ten may include colleagues, neighbors, acquaintances in your community, or even friends you've met through Internet chats who live around the world.

Circle of Ten for Practical and Informational Support

1.
2.
3.
4.
5.
6.

7.
8.
9.
10.

As you list your second Circle of Ten supporters, you may find that your circles overlap, with some of the same people on each list. That's fine. It simply means you have multitalented family or friends!

Personally Speaking

As nutritionists, we want you to keep in mind that food is a great social vehicle. Look for ways to share meals with others, like potluck meals at church, synagogue, or community meetings. Or consider starting an ethnic food club, taking a cooking class, or starting a neighborhood progressive dinner group. For this last, you will need at least four people to participate; everyone goes from one house or apartment to the next for appetizer, salad, entrée, and dessert. It's a fun way to interact using food as the medium.

Step 5: Simplify Your Life

It's no news that another contributor to stress-aging is the degree of complication in our lives today. As we discussed in Chapter 1, time-stacking or juggling two or more activities at the same time is a way of life for millions of us. Yet simplifying our lives is one way we can reduce the clutter and have more personal time for relaxation and enjoyment. In a recent survey in *Health* magazine, 48 percent of the adults surveyed said they have simplified their lives in the last five years.

We can all learn to appreciate simple things in life to make each day better rather than focusing on the negative or the annoying. Try this Circle of Ten Simplifiers to help deactivate stress-aging.

Circle of Ten Simplifiers

1. **Slow down.** Intentionally create times to do nothing but read, listen to music, or sit in the backyard and enjoy nature. You will begin to look forward to this downtime, and life will seem less hectic.
2. **Search for the positive in every situation.** It's no news that negative people are difficult to be around; nothing is ever good enough or fun or right. Positive thinking becomes a habit if you practice it daily. Find something positive to concentrate on even if it's only the weather or the fact that your car is still running.
3. **Listen to or create music.** Research has now documented the positive effects music can have on immunity. Listening to music, singing, or even humming favorite tunes stimulates your brain to release endorphins, chemical messengers that make you feel happy and well. Choose music that is soothing, makes you happy, or helps you to feel relaxed.
4. **Accept change.** There is nothing certain in life except change—so accept this! To help yourself roll with the punches, work on retaining comforting behaviors, like taking an evening stroll, and discard those that are unnecessary, such as ironing sheets or pillowcases.
5. **Increase your confidence.** Develop new skills or increase your knowledge. This will help to improve your view of yourself, as well as improve your performance in all areas of your life.
6. **Exercise your beliefs, and nourish your inner strength.** Explore community service or volunteer work as giving to others will make you feel stronger. If your inner strength

comes from religious faith, spend more time in spiritual activities like prayer or meditation. Take time to enjoy relaxing activities such as walking in the park at sunset, enjoying art or literature, or gardening.

7. **Be responsible.** As you learn to deactivate stress-aging, it's important to be able to make decisions and willingly accept the consequences. As you practice this, you will feel more in control and be more in control. Although some events are outside your sphere, realize that you can have a positive influence on many aspects of life.

8. **Be attentive.** Openly listen to family, friends, and associates, and try to keep up with our rapidly changing world. You will increase your inner confidence if you are in tune with recent developments rather than feeling left behind by change.

9. **Foster hope.** Hope is the central theme to optimism. If you don't believe that things can and will get better, they won't. Negativity and pessimism go hand-in-hand.

10. **Take risks.** People who believe in themselves enough to take risks are the ones who accomplish the most. Be willing to launch out in faith that your idea will work. Again, also be willing to take the consequences, but positive thinking during risk-taking will boost your chances of success.

Step 6: Try Our Circle of Ten Herbs for Optimism and Relaxation

If you have ever downed a cup of hot coffee and realized that it perked you up or allowed you to breathe better, you have tried herbal medicine. Herbal medicine uses natural compounds to treat ailments, such as ginger tea to fight off colds, St. John's Wort to alter moods, or gingko biloba to increase concentration.

According to the World Health Organization (WHO), about

4 billion people or 80 percent of the earth's population uses herbal medicine to receive a desired benefit on the body. Although precise levels of use in the United States are unknown, in 1997, herbal products accounted for sales of more than $3.4 billion, the fastest-growing category in drugstores. Check out the following Circle of Ten Herbs reported to help in improving mood, relieving stress, and deactivating stress-aging.

1. **Chamomile.** This herbal supplement increases relaxation, promotes quality sleep, and can be used to relieve nervousness, upset stomach, and menstrual cramps. Chamomile is available as a dried herb, a supplement, and an herbal tea. A word of caution: Chamomile contains pollen, so it may cause problems for those allergic to ragweed, asters, or chrysanthemums.

2. **Gotu kola.** This herb is native to India, Sri Lanka, South Africa and other tropical climates and has been shown to relieve stress through relaxation. Gotu kola is taken as a capsule or extract.

3. **Ginkgo biloba.** Ginkgo protects cell membranes from free radical damage, improving concentration and memory, increasing blood flow, and helping the symptoms of PMS and depression. It is used to help with short-term memory loss, depression, and other problems of aging. Ginkgo biloba is available in supplements and tea. A word of caution: It may cause nausea, diarrhea, stomach upset, and vomiting in larger doses and reduces clotting time. Anyone taking coumadin should not take this herb. Also, the amount of ginkgo biloba found in herbal tea is probably not effective.

4. **Ginseng.** Ginseng may stimulate the immune response by increasing the number of antibodies in the blood. It is used to stimulate memory, counteract fatigue, and soothe damage caused by stress. Ginseng is available in tea, powder, cap-

sules, tablets, and extract. A word of caution: Ginseng may cause headaches, insomnia, anxiety, breast soreness, or skin rash. More serious side effects include asthma attacks, heart palpations, increased blood pressure or uterine bleeding.
5. **Kava.** Kava is used as a sedative and muscle relaxant. It is a member of the pepper family and has been used in the South Pacific as a natural relaxant. Kava has been reported to help long-term memory, muscle contractibility, insomnia, and anxiety, including the stresses of daily life. Kava is available in tea, tincture, or tablet form. It is recommended that consumption of the active ingredient, kavalactones, be limited to 300 mg per day. A word of caution: High doses of kava can lead to muscle weaknesses, visual impairment, dizziness, and drying or yellowing of the skin. Long-term use of the herb can contribute to hypertension, reduced protein levels, blood cell abnormalities, or liver damage. Therefore, a limit of use for 4 weeks to 3 months is recommended in Australia and required in Germany. Alcohol consumption increases the toxicity of the herb. Do not use if under age 18, pregnant, nursing, or being treated for depression or Parkinson's disease.
6. **Cayenne.** The red fruit of this pepper plant contains capsaicin which works as a pain reliever. Taken in capsules, cayenne can help to relieve migraine or tension headaches. Used as a skin cream or salve, it can relieve chronic pain of arthritis or backaches. Avoid contact with eyes or open wounds, and before using topically, do a skin test for sensitivity.
7. **Passionflower.** This herb is used frequently as a mild tranquilizer and to ease insomnia, stress, and anxiety. Passionflower is available as a tincture, fruit, dried or fresh leaves, or capsules. A word of caution: Be careful not to combine passionflower with prescription sedatives, and do not take if pregnant or nursing.

8. **St. John's Wort.** This herbal supplement is taken to relieve mild depression without some of the common side effects of prescription antidepressants. St. John's Wort is available as capsules, tincture, extract, oil, and dried leaves and flowers. A word of caution: St. John's Wort can cause sensitive skin in sunlight. Check with your doctor if using for depression and do not combine with prescription antidepressants.

9. **Valerian.** Valerian has a sedative effect and has been shown to help in treating insomnia. It is also used to relieve high anxiety, stress, and nervousness. Valerian is available as capsules, tincture, tea, or dried flowers. A word of caution: If you are already taking prescription antidepressants, you should stay away from valerian.

10. **Feverfew.** Researchers have reported that feverfew may inhibit inflammation and act similar to aspirin. Those with stress-related or migraine headaches may be particularly interested in this herb. It is available in supplement form. A word of caution: Anyone with a clotting disorder should consult a physician before taking feverfew.

Just the Facts
Advice About Herbal Therapies

- Herbal and prescription medication interactions do occur. Avoid combined use or ask your pharmacist.
- Lack of standardization and quality control may result in variability in herbal content.
- Herbal treatments should not be used in larger than recommended doses.
- Herbal treatments should not be used continuously for more than several weeks because of a lack of long-term studies.
- Infants, children and the elderly should not use herbal treatments without professional advice.

- Herbal treatments should not be used if contemplating pregnancy, or during pregnancy or lactation.

Journal of the American Medical Association, 11/11/98: 1565-66.

Step 7: Do Mental Aerobics to Stop Stress-Aging

While you are sorting through your Circle of Ten foods, vitamins and supplements, supporters and simplifiers, there is another area we want to share with you: relaxation therapies, or what we call "mental aerobics" that can help you stop stress-aging, reduce anxiety, and even lessen your chances of getting a stress-related illness.

Let's look at some proven ways to unwind or work through stress-related problems that keep you feeling old. (A few can even be done with your spouse, a friend, or someone in your Circle of Ten support group):

- **Art Therapy.** Art therapy is based on human developmental and psychological theories. Using a broad spectrum of creative and artistic methods, the art therapist will help you identify and then change inner emotional conflicts and behavioral problems, as well as help you to increase self-awareness and develop self-esteem. Call your local mental health association for a list of qualified therapists, or enjoy using creative and artistic methods on your own to express your inner feelings.
- **Counseling.** As a rule of thumb, psychological counseling can help most people to develop appropriate coping skills so life's stressors are not as overwhelming. This psychological intervention is an accepted component for everyone—not just the ones who have "psychological problems." Some viable options you may consider include:

1. Individual counseling: A one-on-one session with a therapist in which individual problem areas are addressed. These sessions may include specific help with alleviating depression, anxiety, or stress, along with other personal problem areas.
2. Family counseling: Family members can gather to understand and accept your problems, and the possible impact these may have on your family's lifestyle.
3. Group counseling: Sessions led by trained therapists that allow for the sharing of feelings, as well as the development of effective coping strategies. The exchange of ideas at group sessions is often the most productive way to revamp your thought processes.

- **Dance Therapy.** Using movement, positions, and various postures, the dance therapist helps you to get in touch with your innermost feelings. Once these feelings are brought out and identified, you can move forward in a healthy manner. This form of mind-body treatment is often used with adults who have buried painful memories or those who are too depressed to talk about inner conflicts and resulting emotions.
- **Drama Therapy.** Drama therapy uses drama or theater methods to help you reduce symptoms, integrate the mind and body, or move toward personal growth. Using such techniques as role-play, theater games, mime, puppetry, and improvisation, among many, you can enjoy the creative expression and actually deactivate stress-aging.
- **Meditation.** Meditation is a way of releasing negative thoughts through focusing on a single word or phrase and eliciting the relaxation response. It is recognized as an effective tool in reducing blood pressure, managing chronic pain, and reducing the stress response.
- **Psychotherapy.** Psychotherapy is an effective behavioral treatment that allows you to change your own biology

often in conjunction with prescription medications. Especially for those who obsess on negative thoughts, are highly anxious, or are depressed about their situation in life, psychotherapy helps identify, then verbalize inner conflicts as you learn positive coping skills.

- **Support Groups.** This form of mind-body therapy is geared toward the unique needs of its members, providing both emotional support and education in dealing with illness or life's stressors. While support groups are not psychotherapy groups, they can give you a safe and accepting place to vent frustrations, share personal problems, and receive encouragement from others. The assurance is given that "someone else knows what I am going through," as people share their personal struggles. As shared previously, having a close bond with others is most necessary to revamp your thought processes and feel young again.

Two Down, Four to Go!

There is no "quick fix" for deactivating stress-aging. Sometimes you may feel totally out of control when you are juggling life's interruptions while working and raising children or caring for elderly parents. While you cannot control life's stressors, we've shared with you in Age Deactivator 2 some things you do have control over, and one of the most effective ways to deactivate stress-aging is to change the way you treat yourself and the way you look at life.

As you get these two Age Deactivators under your belt and continue on to Age Deactivator 3—*Let Them Judge You by Your Cover: EAT to Look Young,* we know that you will begin to feel more control in your life. As you will soon experience, this control will soon turn into more energy, greater productivity, and a feeling of being young again!

Age Deactivator 3

Let Them Judge You by Your Cover:

EAT to Look Young

Who would argue that true beauty is more than skin deep? Yet it is no news that how you look surely affects how you feel. When you think you look young, you feel young. And when you feel young, life just seems better. Interestingly, some revealing scientific studies have found that older adults who look attractive and younger than their years also have reduced incidence of illness and more zest for living. How's that for a positive mind-body connection? In this Age Deactivator, we've pulled together some of the best surefire tips on how to guarantee younger looking skin, eyes, and hair—tips you can start using today.

Now that you are "eating your weedies," and have checked your attitude with Age Deactivator 2, it is time to move to the third step in our EAT Plan and start to work on the outer you. No matter how you feel, it is never, ever too late to look young. But before we give you some ways to make this happen, we have some revealing information on how stress-aging affects your skin.

Skin Under Duress

No matter what causes your collision course with stress, it's bound to affect your natural good looks, especially your skin. The reason is cut and dried: When you are stressed, your body focuses on sending blood to your vital organs—the heart, brain, and lungs—rather than to your skin. In simpler terms, that month-long audit at work triggered more than a rapid pulse, insomnia, and a huge accounting bill. It sent stress-aging into high gear, robbing you of your youthful good looks and resulting in pale, ashen skin that makes your undereye circles stand out like a raccoon's eyes.

In addition, when your body is stressed, skin-cell turnover is slowed down, causing that dry, flaky skin. And what about your love affair with a fast-food diet or lack of sleep under stress? All of these factors—a harried lifestyle, poor diet, no sleep, little exercise, and a perpetually tense face—will add up to make you look sallow, pasty, and just plain *old*.

High Anxiety/Damaged Skin

"But I thought skin was just that—skin. Isn't it merely the glue that holds your skeleton together?" Merely the glue? Skin is the largest vital living organ. It's just that while other organs are out of sight, you can actually see the damage stress does to your skin.

Your skin is also multilayered and in a constant state of renewal. Your epidermis (outermost layer of your skin) contains natural moisturizers that help hold water in the skin. With the sun exposure and aging, this outer layer begins to thicken and becomes rougher as fewer cells are replaced when they die. Ever seen a fisherman's face close up? Notice the thickened skin with deep crevices and wrinkles—all resulting from that destructive whammy of sun and age.

Sags, Bags, and Tags

Forget the fisherman, and let's focus on you for now. How would others describe your skin—fresh, sparkling, and glowing? Or draggy, tired, and flaky?

"They could take one look at my skin and say it's turned into sags, bags, and skin tags." Ginah had just lost 20 pounds on a quick weight loss diet, and it was true: her skin looked as if a seamstress needed to take it in on the sides.

Through the years, the elastic fibers that sustain your skin tone also become thicker and less resilient. You may have noticed lately that your skin takes longer to spring back when you pinch it, or it has begun to sag. Part of this responsibility lies with the dermis, which is just below the epidermis or outer layer of skin. The dermis contains sweat glands, hair follicles, blood vessels, nerve endings and the all-important protein fibers, collagen and elastin, which give your skin its backbone. When the collagen and elastin lose their flexibility, your skin will sag, bag, and wrinkle just like old, baggy jeans.

Just the Facts

Experts suggest that 80 percent of skin aging is a result of overexposure to the sun—which of course also plays a major role in skin cancer.

Sun + Time = Partners in Crime

Alicia's problem with old skin was not a result of aging. This 26-year-old woman came to one of our seminars in Florida, seeking the Fountain of Youth for sun-damaged skin, "because I look ancient."

"I've lived in the sun since I was a toddler," Alicia told us. "We had a beach house in Ft. Lauderdale, and every weekend my brothers and I virtually lived on the beach. We ignored sunscreen because we thought our dark tans gave us added protection. Were we wrong! My brother already had a melanoma (skin cancer) removed when he was thirty, and my parents have had basal cell carcinomas (skin cancers) removed from their faces. My skin looks at least ten years older than someone in her mid-twenties.''

Paying the Price for Being Tan

Living in Florida, we've seen the high price people pay for their love affair with the sun. Alicia did have a serious problem, and as we shared with her, now's the time to start living a ''shady life''—literally staying in the shade and out of the sun.

Think of the sun as time's ''partner in crime'' in the aging process. Both sun and aging cause damage to collagen molecules, uncontrolled growth of unhealthy cells such as skin cancer cells, and suppression of the immune system. The sun causes not only wrinkles but also the loss of elasticity in the walls of the tiny blood vessels that feed the skin, which can result in the formation of spider veins. Long-term exposure to the sun can result in cancerous skin cells and some types of serious skin cancers such as *melanoma.*

Researchers suspect that UV B rays are the primary cause of skin cancer, as well as sunburn. UV A rays destroy elastin and collagen over time, which leads to aging and may also cause sunburn and skin cancer.

Weather forecasters rank the day's level of ultraviolet radiation in numbers from 1 to 15. Anything above 8 means you'd better be wearing sunglasses and plenty of sunscreen the entire time you are out. According to dermatologist Albert Kligman and biologist Lorraine Kligman, unprotected skin allows the UV radiation to prematurely wrinkle your skin as well as causing mutations (abnormal changes) in your cells. This process sets you up for skin cancer a few years down the road. Staying out of the sun not only stops wrinkles and cancers from developing, but it lets your skin do some much needed repair work on itself.

Red Alert
If you are going to be outdoors, try to avoid the sun's strongest hours of 10:00 A.M. till 2:00 P.M.

Blocking Those Rays

Unfortunately, when Alicia was a child, she missed the benefit of sunscreen. Nonetheless, her children can take advantage of this protection starting at an early age. Most dermatologists suggest that you use a sunscreen with a Sun Protection Factor (SPF) of at least 15 and reapply about every 2 hours. If you live or spend time in a southern region or have fair skin, choose sun products with an SPF of at least 20, preferably 30, and apply hourly or as often as it takes to prevent your skin from turning that light pink color.

Most sunscreen products contain chemicals that protect skin by absorbing the UV light and then causing it to dissipate. In order for these products to protect you, they need to be applied about 30 minutes before you hit the outdoors.

Sun Damage or Life Damage?

"Sun damage? What about life damage? I swear, just living in the world is enough to make me look old." Our friend Sarah may have coined a new term with "life damage," but isn't it true? Think about what your body is going through from the ravages of stress and time. We're the first to assert that "laugh lines" are *not* funny. Combined with increasing grooves in the forehead, drooping eyelids, sallow skin, and drab, diminished hair, is it any wonder that alpha-hydroxy acid (AHA) beauty products took in more than $300 million their first three years on the market?

What about the rising incidence of plastic surgery? In 1992, 41 percent of all elective plastic surgery was performed on 35- to 50-year-olds of both sexes—procedures that barely existed twenty years ago. Although the use of cosmetics has greatly declined among 18- to 29-year-olds, women aged 30 to 59 now use more cosmetics than their counterparts did 6 years ago. As one client complained before she began the EAT Plan, "Now that I'm forty, it takes me twice as long to look half as good as I used to."

Yes, although time is not on your side when it comes to having younger-looking skin, there are some exciting things you can do to revitalize your skin and *save face*—no matter how old you are and how much stress or sun you've had. We want you to follow the six steps in Age Deactivator 3, and see if someone in the next few weeks doesn't stop you on the street to say how marvelous you look.

Step 1: Eat to Rejuvenate Your Skin

Because this is the EAT Plan, it's only natural that the first step in Age Deactivator 3 is to eat a diet rich in antioxidant-loaded foods. Remember that antioxidants are naturally occurring compounds in foods that attack free radicals in your body and destroy them. A host of scientific studies have found that these foods may help protect your skin against skin cancer and photo-aging (damage from sunlight). As you read in Chapter 3 and Age Deactivator 1, foods containing beta-carotene, vitamin C, selenium, vitamin E, and calcium are all part of the EAT Plan. Taking a supplement (page 65) is also a wise move as many people, especially women, do not get enough of these much-needed vitamins and minerals.

While you may not think of calcium as a key player in skin care, it is important for preventing wrinkles. You also need calcium for keeping your bones strong and healthy. Not only does bone loss (osteoporosis) lead to painful and disfiguring fractures, but it can lead to skin that sags just like that old pair of jeans. Just as vitamin C aids in the production of collagen, calcium helps every bone maintain its density and keeps you standing tall—pulling all that loose skin tightly over your skeleton to keep it smooth.

Twenty-five Bone Builders

Skim and low-fat milk
Nonfat and low-fat yogurt
Ice cream
Sherbet
Buttermilk
Cheese
Cottage cheese
Ricotta cheese
Evaporated skim milk
Nonfat milk powder
Calcium-fortified orange juice
Calcium-enriched bread
Calcium-fortified cereal
Macaroni and cheese
White beans
Salmon with bones
Sardines with bones
Spinach
Turnip greens
Bok choy
Curly endive
Pudding
Nonfat cream cheese
Tofu (check label for calcium content)
Calcium-fortified soy milk

Think Zinc!

A recent study from the U.S. Department of Agriculture's Human Nutrition Research Center on Aging at Tufts University found that when you increase your calcium intake, there appears to be a severe reduction in zinc absorption. Zinc is critically important for proper functioning of the immune system. This does not mean we need to cut our calcium intake, but it does mean that we need to make sure we are also getting enough zinc, since many typical American diets fall short. A standard vitamin-mineral supplement should provide you with all the needed zinc but here are some zinc superstars that may also help.

Zinc Superstars

Oysters, shellfish, and other seafood	Eggs
Lean red meat	Fortified cereals
Lean pork	Baked beans
Chicken	Low-fat milk and yogurt
Turkey	Tofu

Lower Fat = Lower Risk of Skin Cancer

In addition to a diet loaded with antioxidant-rich foods, there is some compelling evidence that a low-fat diet (20 percent of calories from fat) may help prevent some forms of skin cancer. Researchers at Baylor College of Medicine in Houston studied skin-cancer patients on both a low-fat diet (20 percent fat) and a control group diet (38 percent fat). After evaluating the patients every 4 months for 2 years, the patients in the high-fat diet group were 5 times more likely to have premalignant lesions which can lead to cancerous tumors. Though researchers are not sure why a low-fat diet may protect the skin, one suspicion is that a healthy diet (that is, a diet filled with loads of fruits and vegetables) boosts the immune system in its war against the production of harmful cells.

Twenty-five Skin Savers

If the combined ravages of sun and stress make you look like Whistler's mother, then stop your fretting, and keep eating! The following Skin Savers are your prescription to help protect against skin cancer, photoaging, and wrinkles, as they are loaded with antioxidants, phytochemicals, protein, etc. Notice that the fruit and vegetables are deeply colored with orange, yellow, and green, signs of antioxidant and phytochemical content. All of these foods are in Age Deactivator 1 as options for your Circle of Ten foods:

Apricots	Oranges
Peaches	Cranberries
Nectarines	Berries
Kiwi	Melon
Papaya	Fish
Mango	Garlic
Carrots	Eggs
Red and green peppers	Chicken
Sweet potatoes	Seeds
Broccoli	Nuts
Spinach	Avocado
Cantaloupe	Low-fat dairy products
Garlic	

Just the Facts

Certain beverages can also provide phytochemical and anti-oxidant benefits. Researchers at the University of Kansas have found that black, green, and oolong teas contain a strong antioxidant substance (polyphenol) that may provide benefits to the body as great as vitamins E and C. Green tea is more delicate than black or oolong and requires only 1 to 1½ minutes of brewing. Black and oolong tea need 3 to 5 minutes for full, robust flavor. In most cases, the decaffeination process does not remove the antioxidants. Herbal tea is not actually tea but a combination of flowers, roots, plant leaves, and spices. They typically do not contain caffeine unless they have been blended with regular tea.

Step 2: Start Your Sun-Damage Reversal Routine

While the best remedy for younger-looking skin is never, ever have unprotected contact with the sun, most of us are far beyond that point. Especially during our teenage years, when being tan was equated with being healthy, most of us looked "really healthy." Remember lathering on coconut oil or a mixture of baby oil and iodine, then lying on a beach blanket for hours just waiting for the sun to brown us? Yes, sun damage has already taken its toll.

Yet no matter how damaged your skin is, you can help reverse some of this by using the following Sun-Smart Strategies:

1. *Wear sunscreen daily.* (Remember to protect often neglected areas that get the most sun exposure such as the eyes, face, neck, and the backs of your hands.

2. *Use a product that protects against both UVA and UVB ultraviolet light, such as zinc oxide.* Look for products containing Z-Cote, a transparent form of zinc oxide or avobenzone (or known as Parsol 1789). Products containing

titanium dioxide are also available for those who can't wait and need impromptu protection; these products take effect immediately.

3. *Use a sunscreen with an SPF (sun protection factor) of 15 or above.*

4. *Stay out of the sun from 10:00 A.M. till 2:00 P.M. when the UV rays are the strongest.* By doing so, you can reduce your UV exposure by as much as 80 percent annually.

5. *Always wear a hat when you are in the sun.*

6. *Wear sunglasses that offer UV protection.* (Choose sunglasses that protect from both UVA and UVB rays, and look for glasses with a wraparound style.)

7. *Wear a T-shirt over sunscreen for more protection (darker is better).*

8. *Use a sunless tanning product if you want the look of a tan.*

Lingo Lowdown

The SPF (sun protection factor) rating refers only to UVB rays. The SPF number tells you the percentage of sun rays blocked by the sunscreen. An SPF of 15 lets 1 ray of sunlight in 15 hit your skin, a protection rate of 93 percent, while SPF 30 allows 1 in 30 rays to reach your skin, for a protection of 97 percent. Make sure your product protects for both UVA and UVB rays.

Now, Wear Your Weedies

Now research also suggests that wearing your vitamins A, C, and E is as important as eating them. While most of us are aware that antioxidants fight heart disease and cancer, researchers now assert that these nutritional goldmines also attack wrinkles.

Dermatologist and researcher Serge Hercberg, M.D., Ph.D., national coordinator of the SUVIMAX (Supplementation, Vitamin and Mineral, and Antioxidant) trial, suggests that applying antioxidant vitamins and minerals to the skin may reduce long-term damage caused by environmental exposure and promote self-repair of existing damage. In other words, the abuse to our skin from those years of "spring break" tans may be somewhat repaired.

Call for Damage Control

As much as you try to protect your skin, most active people have at least one mild sunburn each year or two. Here are answers to your call for damage control:

- Take two aspirin tablets every 6 hours to reduce inflammation over the first 24 hours.
- Use cool compresses of water, tea, aloe, or milk for 10 minutes at a time.
- Smooth on aloe vera gel or aloe straight from the plant. Pierce a piece of the plant to obtain the gel.
- Apply topical hydrocortisone cream to help reduce swelling.

Red Flag

Some drugs (both over-the-counter and prescription) can cause you to be sun-sensitive. Some of these include oral contraceptives, antihistamines, coal-tar shampoo, tetracycline, and sulfa drugs. Skin creams such as Retin-A or Renova also cause sun sensitivity. Check with your pharmacist if you are uncertain.

Step 3: Use Antiaging Products to Revitalize Your Skin

If you are already showing a few lines (well, maybe more than a few!) from life's more tumultuous experiences, there are some excellent revitalizing skin products you can try. These are scientifically proven to help smooth some of those fine lines and reduce the appearance of wrinkles.

Lingo Lowdown

There are two types of wrinkles: fine and dynamic folds. *Fine wrinkles* are there all the time; *dynamic folds* (wrinkles) are like forehead wrinkles and smile lines that extend from your nose to your mouth that become more prominent when you laugh or speak. Personally speaking, we don't think wrinkles are either *fine* or *dynamic,* do you?

Just the Facts

Try these quick-and-easy beverages to hydrate your skin and keep it supple:

- Bottled water
- Carbonated water
- Mineral water
- Tap water

The Latest in Skin Savers

With such a diverse selection of skin products, it's not easy to know which ones are best for your skin. While a trip to the dermatologist might be a wise investment, as this doctor can answer questions pertinent to your situation, here is an overview of the top products in the market:

- *Retin-A* and *Renova* are prescription formulations based on the active ingredient tretinoin, a family member of vitamin A. Tretinoin works to slough off dead surface cells, thicken the skin's healthy cells, and increase the production of collagen. All of these benefits make the skin appear more supple and less wrinkled (now that's when we think our skin looks *fine* and *dynamic!*). Within 12 to 14 weeks of use, your fine lines should have diminished, and there should be noticeable improvement in age spots, discoloration, and rough patches. Renova and Retin-A have been through rigorous FDA testing and are available only through a prescription.

- *Alpha-hydroxy acids* (AHAs) are made from natural substances such as glycolic acid (from sugar cane) and lactic acid (from sour milk). They are used topically to slough off dead cells, forcing new cells (and youthful-looking skin) to replace them. Some dermatologists suggest that regular use of AHAs can subtly help fade age spots, lessen fine lines, and soften rough patches. Remember, these products don't prevent skin damage, they just work to improve the skin you have now.

You can buy AHAs at your local drugstore. Dermatologists use much stronger treatments in their office with solutions of 20 to 70 percent, whereas over-the-counter products contain only 2 to 12 percent.

Red Flag

AHAs, Renova, and Retin-A can increase your sensitivity to the sun and cause skin irritation. Start with a product containing a mild concentration and work your way up. Carefully follow directions for use on the package.

- *Beta-hydroxy* acids are mild acids like alpha-hydroxy that dislodge debris from the bottom of pores so that they may possibly return to normal size. BHAs usually don't cause irritation or sun sensitivity. A combination of BHA-AHA may bring you the best of both ingredients.

- *ERT (estrogen replacement therapy)* is yet another skin saver for women at menopause or for those who have had early menopause owing to a hysterectomy and removal of the ovaries. Rodolphe Maheux, Chairman of the Department of Obstetrics and Gynecology at Laval University, in Quebec City, Canada, has found that estrogen replacement therapy after menopause preserves not just bone but also skin. This is because collagen, a building block of skin, is slowly eroded along with the declining estrogen level associated with menopause. Women lose an estimated 30 milligrams of collagen from the skin daily, resulting in thinner, dryer skin that starts to look like plastic wrap. Maheux found that women increased the thickness of their skin by 12 percent after taking estrogen for 1 year.

- *Vitamin C creams* (about 8 percent concentration) may decrease discoloration of the skin and may help repair sun-induced skin damage by destroying free radicals. Some test tube studies suggest that these creams may speed up the production of collagen, but the jury is still out.

- *Retinol lotions* are similar to the prescription products Retin-A and Renova but are less potent, so they may achieve a similar result over a longer period of time. Retinol is a member of the vitamin A family that is involved in making collagen and elastin; with age, the level of retinol in the skin decreases.

- *Prescription cocktails* may also give your aging skin a youthful glow. Studies show that skin discoloration can be reduced with a combination of Retin-A, vitamin C, 10 percent glycolic acid, and 4 to 8 percent hydroquinone. Ask your dermatologist about this prescription cocktail to see if it would help in your situation.

- *Salicyclic acid* is a member of the beta-hydroxy family. This FDA-approved acne medication is now being added to moisturizing products and is great for cleaning out oil and dirt from the pores, which is the root cause of acne.
- *Facial compresses* are now available that hydrate and moisturize the skin. In some cases, these compresses make skin firmer for just a couple of hours.
- *Firming serums* are also available that contain substances called polymers that feel like a film and tighten the face temporarily, just like support hose. There are also enzyme exfoliators that use bromelain or papain (enzymes found in pineapple and papayas).
- *Firming gel masks* remove blackheads and oil near the surface when the masks harden and are peeled off. Your pores will appear smaller for a few days after this gel application.
- *Adhesive strips* are similar to gel masks in that they stick to the debris that clogs your pores and pull it out. These strips are available over-the-counter and have been found to remove some blackheads.
- *Firming eye gels* tighten the skin temporarily and help disperse fluid with natural ingredients such as aloe and cucumber.

Red Flag

Before you try a new skin product, rub a small amount on your arm and watch it for 24-hours to make sure you are not allergic to it.

Nip and Tuck

What if these products are not enough to do what you want? In 1997 more than 2 million Americans underwent cosmetic surgery or nonsurgical cosmetic procedures, according to the

American Society for Aesthetic Plastic Surgery (ASAPS). The most common procedures performed were chemical peels, collagen injections, liposuction, eyelid surgery, and laser skin resurfacing. The top three procedures for men, who accounted for 14 percent of these cosmetic surgeries, were hair transplantation, nose reshaping, and liposuction. Baby boomers (35 to 50) had 46 percent of all the cosmetic procedures performed. About 24 percent of procedures were for people ages 19 to 34, and 22 percent for ages 51 to 64.

Just the Facts

Before you elect plastic surgery, be sure to:

- Look at the doctor's credentials, particularly a certification or board eligibility from the American Board of Plastic Surgery.
- Look for an affiliation with a hospital.
- Get several opinions.
- Ask for referrals and see before-and-after photographs of clients.
- Ask about the plastic surgeon's experience with the procedure you want.
- Be thoroughly educated—read, read, read!

Zapped by the Light

Carbon dioxide lasers to zap wrinkles sounds like something out of a science fiction novel, but over the last few years this treatment, known as laser peel, laser resurfacing, or laser exfoliation, is rapidly becoming an effective, minimally invasive way of treating certain types of wrinkles. It delivers a high burst of laser light in a very short period of time (a millisecond), and the depth to which it penetrates the skin can be controlled to reduce the potential for burning and scarring. The laser vaporizes the outer wrinkled layer of skin, allowing the new layer underneath to regenerate. Laser surgery can be effective on "lipstick bleed," that area around the lips where there are fine wrinkles. It can also make the skin more prone to dark spots (hyperpigmentation), so a sunscreen with an SPF of 15 or more should be worn when outside. Other tools dermatologists use for fighting wrinkles include chemical peeling and dermabrasion. Dermabrasion uses a sandpaper-like disk to remove the outer layer of skin, while chemical peels use glycolic and other stronger chemicals to remove cells.

Pump It Up!

Collagen injections are used to fill up wrinkled skin. Your physician will want to make sure you are not allergic to collagen, and since it tends to dissolve, the procedure usually needs to be redone every 6 months.

Another new treatment is *isolage,* in which your doctor sends a small piece of your skin to the lab, and it returns in an injectable form used in place of collagen. There is no chance you'll be allergic to it and it reportedly lasts longer.

Red Flag

Some things that won't help:

Facial massage and electronic facial machines may feel good but they will do nothing more than temporarily boost your circulation and work moisturizer into the skin; they don't fight wrinkles.

Astringents and home steaming do not minimize pores. Astringents that contain alcohol tighten pores only for a few minutes, while steaming loosens the particles in the pores but doesn't dislodge them.

Step 4: Take Care of Unsightly Problems

Just when your face starts to look younger, you look down at your thighs and calves and see bulging and unsightly veins. Isn't it amazing how something so seemingly harmless can look so awful?

A varicose vein is a twisted, enlarged vein (blood vessel that returns blood back to the heart) that usually occurs near the skin surface. They are different from spider veins, which are usually very fine and cause only superficial discoloring. When the valves that normally keep blood moving toward the heart and prevent backflow no longer work properly, blood flows backward and pools form in the veins. Physicians think that varicose veins run in families, although pregnancy, obesity, lack of exercise, and regular, prolonged sitting or standing (in one place) may all play a part. Varicose veins may cause no discomfort or may ache and even cause fluid retention or edema near the ankles and problems with blood flow.

There are many treatment options for varicose veins. Depending on the severity of your problem, you could choose from the following:

- Camouflage cosmetics
- Support hose (light-support) in fashion colors
- A mild pain reliever like acetaminophen or aspirin (check with your doctor or health care provider)
- Avoiding standing or sitting for long periods of time without flexing your ankles or moving around some
- Sclerotherapy, or injection of a chemical to cause withering of the varicose vein
- Surgical removal of veins

While varicose veins are usually not serious, see your doctor to make sure. Don't second guess the severity of your problem.

Don't Date Yourself

Other than varicose veins, there are other unsightly problems you may have that you do not need to live with. Check out the list to see which problems you need to take care of:

- Dark leathery skin from too much sun
- Dated hairstyles
- Split ends
- Drab gray hair
- Too much foundation
- Dated makeup and fashions
- Heavy, dark eye makeup
- Hair growing on face (women)
- Long hairs peeping out of nose and ears
- Skin tags or unsightly moles that can be removed
- Poor dental care and stained teeth
- Dark undereye circles from lack of sleep
- Dry, scaly skin from lack of moisturizing

Step 5: Protect Those Tresses From Daily Stresses

When stress-aging is activated, even your hair will look old. But you can stop a bad hair day quickly by using herbal infusions. For centuries, herbal infusions have been used as rinses to revitalize hair. To make your own infusion, steep ¼ cup of one of the following fresh or dried herbs in 3 cups of water for 12 minutes. Cool, strain, and use as a final rinse.

You might try:

- Chamomile—to add gloss and highlights to light brown and blonde hair.
- Ginseng—to replenish moisture, add sheen, and give hair flexibility.

- Lavender—to renew hair's shine and silkiness.
- Lemon grass—to condition hair and make it shine.
- Rosemary—to help hair grow and control dandruff.

Red Flag
If you are allergic to ragweed, be wary of products that contain chamomile, which is a relative of ragweed. It can cause some of the same symptoms such as a runny nose, headaches, congestion, or itchy eyes.

But I Have No Tresses!

Hair loss is one side effect of stress-aging that is not pretty. Simply put, hair loss is an abnormal loss of hair from the face or scalp. Sometimes hair loss results from a poor diet, infections of the scalp, internal organ disease, hormonal changes such as pregnancy or menopause, or aging, but stress is also a big culprit.

What are the symptoms? Thinning of the hair, or patchy loss of hair over the scalp and other hair-bearing areas such as the beard (for men) or eyebrows. While it is normal to lose 50 to 100 hairs a day, hair loss becomes abnormal if you begin to lose more than 100 hairs a day.

There are three kinds of hair loss:

Androgenetic alopecia, or male pattern baldness: Can affect both men and women and runs in families.

Alopecia areata, or loss of hair in clumps: Has no known cause, although it is speculated to be an autoimmune disease that can run in families.

Telogen Effluvium: Usually occurs a few months following childbirth or from an acute illness, fever, physical or emotional stress, or improper diet.

Red Alert

Forget brushing your hair 100 times a night as that may actually pull your hair out. Avoid hair products such as strong lotions, perms, and dyes that can damage or break your hair. Keep your hormones in check as this can influence hair loss, and make sure your diet has ample protein.

Growing New Hair

There are several products available now to treat hair loss. One over-the-counter product, minoxidil (Rogaine), may help to make thinning hair look fuller, but this new hair is lost if the treatment is stopped. At $30 to $40 for one month's supply, this is a costly investment for only temporary results. There is some evidence that finasteride (Proscar), a treatment for prostate problems, may stimulate hair growth, and another new prescription drug, Propecia, has also been used with some good results.

Yet none of these new remedies is a guarantee of a new head of hair. Not even hair transplantation—transplanting small plugs of hair one hair at a time—is foolproof. If new growth does occur, it will happen in 1 to 3 months (at a healthy $15,000 for a complete scalp!).

Custom hair pieces are also an option. Check with the American Hair Loss Council for assistance.

Step 6: Try Natural Recipes for Soothing Skin Care

Sometimes the best way to pamper skin is the natural way. Check out our natural home remedies for problems associated with stress-aging:

Beauty Problem	Natural Remedy
Tired, puffy eyes	• Tea bags. The tannin in tea helps reduce puffiness. Tea bags should be steeped and then cooled. • Frozen gel masks. Put in your freezer, cover eyes for 5 to 10 minutes. The cold contracts the tissue. • Decrease your salt (sodium) intake for a week or two and see if it helps with water retention. • Antihistamines can often help undereye puffiness if it is caused by allergies, but check with your health care professional. • Sleep with your head slightly elevated.
Dry, tired skin	• Soak a face cloth in a mixture of equal parts water and milk (low-fat or skim is fine). Place on face or other body parts for 10 minutes and then rinse. • Oatmeal mask or scrub. It soothes and softens skin as well as draws out impurities. • Papaya mask or scrub. The papain enzyme helps slough off dead skin cells. • Aloe vera gel. This is soothing, healing, and hydrates the skin without oil. Use the gel or a leaf from a plant (slice open to extract the gel inside). • Cucumber juice. Has a soothing effect on oily and blemished skin. • Honey. It coats the skin with a film that helps it to rehydrate itself. Often used in a mask with yogurt.

Just the Facts
Superfatted soaps like Dove or Basis or glycerine bars like Neutrogena help minimize moisture loss in the shower. Since water is the skin's primary source of moisture, most treatments for dry skin are aimed at adding it to or trapping it in the epidermis.

Red Flag

If you use a loofah when you shower or bathe, be sure that it dries thoroughly between uses and that every couple of weeks you soak it in a solution of one part bleach to ten parts water. Bacteria can thrive in this wet environment and cause rashlike conditions on your skin.

Just the Facts

Did you know?

- Moisturizers work best when applied to wet skin, such as right after bathing.
- For tired, achy feet, try a soak in your favorite bubble bath mixed with Epsom salts in warm water.

Just 10 Minutes a Day

If you will pledge to give 10 minutes each day to improve the "outer you," you can be well on your way to younger looking skin and hair. Try the following 10-minute remedies for skin, hair, hands, and feet:

10 Minutes to Fancy Feet

Spas aren't the only ones with secrets to pampered feet. Mix your favorite body cream with baking soda to make a thick paste. Rub all over your feet, remembering not to neglect your heels and soles, then rinse. Gently rub a pumice stone or tool designed for the feet over any rough areas. Next, apply a layer of petroleum jelly or oil such as olive and put on a pair of cotton socks. Sleep in the socks or put up your feet for a few minutes and let the oil do its magic.

10 Minutes to Satiny-Soft Hands

Since hands are a surefire giveaway for your age, give them an occasional facial. Next time you do the dishes or your delicate lingerie, coat your hands with your favorite hand cream or petroleum jelly, then put on your rubber gloves. The heat from the water will aid the cream in softening your hands. Now that was quick and easy!

Try coating your hands with honey, and then massage them with powdery ground oatmeal for a couple of minutes. Wash your hands and then apply hand cream or petroleum jelly, and slip on a pair of cotton gloves for 10 minutes or longer. The difference will be impressive!

10 Minutes to Soft, Shiny Hair

If your hair feels dry and looks dull, check out our Kitchen Cures. Coat dry hair with mayonnaise or olive oil (other oils such as canola work fine), wrap head with plastic wrap followed by a warm towel, and relax for 10 minutes or longer with your favorite book. Shampoo out with an herbal shampoo for a great feel and smell.

10 Minutes to Smoother Skin

To make a pampering facial scrub, mix baking soda with a cleanser such as Cetaphil or Aquanil to form a paste and gently rub into skin. Rinse with cool water and pat dry. Other mixtures that work well as a paste include finely ground oats (fine as baby powder) mixed with the cleansers above or water and ground dried beans (ground very fine) mixed with above cleansers or water.

Go Ahead and Let 'Em Guess

Remember the woman who said it took her twice as long to look half as good as she used to? If that's the case, then she needs to fine-tune her beauty routine. If you are spending more than 30 to 45 minutes getting yourself together—shower, hair, face—then your beauty routine is way too complicated.

We asked John Soper, makeup specialist and owner of Blades Hair Salon in Orlando, Florida, to tell us the top ten secrets to destress and quickly rejuvenate tired skin:

1. Cleanse and moisturize (while skin is damp) eye area and face with products containing AHAs.
2. Gently cleanse face and then relax for 10 minutes with slices of cucumber on your eyes and a cloth soaked in ice-cold milk on your face. You can wash your face with cold milk if you prefer.
3. For a quick pick-me-up, cleanse your face, then gently put your face in a sink filled with ice. Or use ice packs on the eyes and face.
4. Use a firming gel for bags under the eyes.
5. Use concealer at the outside corner of the eyes to perk them up.
6. Use concealer in the folds from the corner of the nose to the corner of the mouth.
7. Remember that less is more when it comes to makeup. It's the application, not the amount, of makeup that enhances your natural beauty.
8. Stay with neutral colors for the lips, eyes, and cheeks.
9. Use shades of brown for eyeliner instead of black to avoid harshness and drawing attention to tired eyes.
10. Avoid gray and the red family of eye shadows. These make you look tired and older, especially when you feel

tired. The same holds true for highly frosted shadows—choose matte finishes instead.

Sweet Dreams

As you finish Age Deactivator 3, there are still a few more gentle steps you can take each night to slow down the passage of time while you are sleeping:

1. Use a lip conditioner.
2. Apply a super-rich cream to hands.
3. Sleep on a satin pillowcase.
4. Moisturize feet with an AHA lotion and sleep in socks.
5. Coat your body with lotion (containing AHAs if desired).
6. Put a tad of conditioner (like petroleum jelly) on lashes.
7. Use eye cream or gel.
8. Massage face and throat with cream/lotion.

Remember our friend Sarah, who said she looked older simply because of "life's damage"? Now that she has all the knowledge needed to look young again, Sarah has been working hard to put these six steps into practice, and wow, what a difference!

Now don't close the book, thinking you've got all the answers. You still have only half the plan. There are three more Age Deactivators to go—and plenty of innovative and scientifically proven ideas that will keep you looking and feeling young. So, move on to Age Deactivator 4 and keep that momentum going.

Get Your Buns off the Back Burner:

EAT to Stay Strong and Stand Tall

When Gayle, now 39, came to our stress-aging seminar several years ago, she could barely walk up the auditorium stairs without pausing to catch her breath. More than 25 pounds overweight, this once-attractive woman was a star athlete in high school and college, swimming the 500-yard freestyle. Yet after college Gayle started a sedentary career as a computer analyst, then had three babies within a 4-year period.

"I'm too old for my age," Gayle told us. "Not only do I feel lethargic and tired, but look at me! I'm fat, frumpy, and look old enough to be the grandmother, not the mother of three children."

Gayle went on to tell how exercise was not at all a part of her life. "Exercise? Are you kidding? I can barely move around to get my housework done without getting short of breath. Then, it seems the less I move, the more weight I gain. The heavier I get, the harder it is to move at all. I just want to enjoy my children like other moms."

Gayle's plea for help in regaining her youthful vitality and good looks is common. In an informal survey of more than 1,000 of our seminar participants, 900 or 90 percent said to look and feel young was important in all aspects of life—at home, work, or play.

Obviously, if you have hit 30, you know that time is no longer on your side! Think about it. Compared with the carefree days of childhood spent gazing at clouds or swinging for hours at the nearby park, now the clock calculates everything you do. From dashing out the door with a cup of coffee in hand to make your office car pool, to rushing to meet client deadlines, to juggling child raising with after-school activities and community volunteering—time is a much-valued commodity. Most of us feel like our colleague Sam, who admitted that after all the time in his day was spent meeting the needs of others, there was only a handful of change, or "mere minutes," left for himself.

Knowing that most of us usually run out of time before we ever run out of money, we believe that this fourth step in the EAT Plan, "Get Your Buns off the Back Burner: EAT to Stay Strong and Stand Tall," must be quick, efficient, and show amazingly *fast* results to keep you motivated. With Age Deactivator 4, we will give you the perfect ℞ to feeling young with 5- to 10-minute doses of activity and movement, and all in just four easy steps.

Streamlining That Million-Dollar Racehorse

No matter what shape you're in, it's crucial to love yourself. In Age Deactivator 1, we compared your body to a highly valued Mercedes-Benz. Now we want you to see how your body is also designed to be as efficient as a million-dollar racehorse, as it is built to run at its peak. To get the peak performance benefit, in this Age Deactivator we want you to incorporate a variety of daily exercises, including:

- Stretching
- Walking or other aerobic activity
- Enjoyable activities such as gardening or playing with the kids
- Weight lifting or resistance training, including using machines, rubber bands, or even canned foods from the pantry, every two to three days

---

Just the Facts

If you have arthritis, you will probably benefit from exercise, particularly weight lifting. A study conducted at Tufts University found that people with rheumatoid arthritis could safely increase their strength by up to 60 percent with a modest training program. Another study published in the *Journal of the American Medical Association* also found improvements in osteoarthritis when patients combined weight training with aerobic exercise. To gain the strengthening benefit without irritating the joints, proper technique is important. Be sure to check with your physician, then consult with a physical therapist so that you have a program planned with your special needs in mind.

Step 1: Make Sure You Can Take the Heat

As you begin Age Deactivator 4, we want to make sure you are healthy enough to get those buns moving without any problems. We're talking about feeling younger—and being an invalid after a sports injury is not in our plan!

If you are a woman under 50 or a man under 40 and in good health, there is probably no need for physician involvement with a moderate exercise program. However, if you are older than this and haven't been active for a while, or if you answer yes to any of the following questions, at any age, the American College of Sports Medicine (ACSM) recommends that you see your physician or health care provider before you begin.

1. Are you a diabetic?
2. Have you ever had chest pain during physical activity?
3. Do you have any joint or bone problems?
4. Do you have asthma or other breathing problems?
5. Are you pregnant?
6. Do you have hypertension (high blood pressure)?
7. Do you have a heart condition?
8. Do you take any heart or blood pressure medications?
9. Do you ever feel dizzy?
10. Do you have any other medical condition that could interfere with exercise?

If you do have concerns about your health or if you just want to make sure you are in tip-top shape, go ahead and ask your doctor for a physical evaluation.

Step 2: Become Your Own Personal Trainer

Remember Sam, who said that if there was any time left each day, it was just like a "handful of change" to him? We know your schedule is tight, but we also believe that making time to exercise can be a priceless investment in your health, especially when you consider how it zaps stress-aging. That's why it's important for you to make exercise happen.

"But I hate to exercise," you say. We know. Millions of people do. Yet we think we know why people hate to exercise, and it's very simple: Exercise has become complicated, confusing, and quite honestly, inconvenient. That's why we believe the fastest and easiest way to get in shape is to become your own personal trainer, and that's a breeze, if you follow our Circle of Ten exercise tips. Check out the following tips we use, both personally and with clients:

Tip 1: Set personal goals. Using your personal training diary (an inexpensive three-ringed notebook, a section in your calendar, or whatever works for you), set realistic goals for each week. In other words, a goal such as "I will lose 20 pounds by Thanksgiving" is unrealistic and almost always destined for failure. We want you to use bite-size realistic goals. For example, you may write in your personal training diary: "This week I will add a fun activity such as walking the mall or playing tennis to my schedule." Now that goal is one most of us can accomplish.

Once you've set your exercise goal for the week, you have to consider how you are going to find time to accomplish it. That's where a calendar comes in handy. Look ahead at the upcoming week for you and your family. Where could you squeeze in exercise? Perhaps you could walk in the mall while the kids are at gymnastics nearby. Maybe you could play tennis early Saturday morning before family commitments face you. Or you might try setting your alarm for 30 minutes earlier each day and walking the dog before making breakfast and getting everyone off to work and school. One woman we know keeps her rollerblades in the trunk of her car. When she drops her children off at piano or dance lessons, she spends the waiting time in-line skating in that particular neighborhood.

Think about what works for you, then pencil in the time, place, and specific activity or exercise. Making exercise a structured part of your life will let it happen much easier.

Tip 2: Choose activities that have your name on them. Remember, convenience is crucial. If it isn't convenient for you, you most likely aren't going to do it. Which reminds us, backyard benefits count, too. Be sure to include family games like basketball, badminton, soccer, and jump rope, as well as much-needed chores such as leaf raking, wood chopping or splitting, active gardening, window washing, and grass cutting. Ever heard of

using soup cans or a bicycle tube for a workout? The sky's the
limit when it comes to fun, effective ways to exercise.

Red Flag

Consider consulting with a physical therapist or an American
College of Sports Medicine certified exercise specialist, if
needed, to find which exercises are best for your body and for
what you are trying to achieve. It's better to know proper form
ahead of time than deal with aches and pains from a sports
injury.

Stretch This Way

We have heard stretching called the "Rodney Dangerfield of
Exercise." Why? Because it don't get no respect! Have you ever
noticed how a cat stretches throughout the day, particularly upon
waking. We can learn from them. Scientist Abby King of the
Stanford Medical School says that stretching not only improves
circulation to the muscles and joints, but increases your range of
motion so that movement is easier. Stretching helps to alleviate
aches and pains like creaky knees and stiff backs. For those with
arthritis, stretching helps your body have full range of motion.

No matter what your age or which activities you choose,
always start out by stretching your body to warm it up.

Diversify Your Workout

If walking is your main form of exercise, you may want to
consider *fartlek,* also known as speed play, in your routine. For
example, walk for 2 to 3 minutes, then run for 2 to 3 minutes,
then repeat the cycle again and again. You're not the only one

who has difficulty working your body for 20 minutes at a high intensity, so short bursts of intensity can help make a difference. Fartlek can also give you the intensity without the feeling of burnout or putting your body at risk for injury. Try to add a hill or steps to your next walk, or run between a few telephone poles or road signs.

Just Walk On By

By the way, if you are a walker, have you tried heel-to-toe walking? This megaform of walking uses your entire body and requires a bit more out of you than regular walking but is well worth the effort and benefits. Not only is it great for toning your muscles (especially those in the buttocks, waist, hips, and thighs), but it's an amazing way to tone flabby arms. While the official name is *racewalking,* we prefer the original name: heel-to-toe walking. After all, Age Deactivator 4 is *not* about beating someone in a race—the one thing you're trying *not* to do as you deactivate stress-aging! Rather, we want you to move more or walk in such a way as to achieve a maximum whole body workout and enjoy it at the same time. This is *not* an oxymoron, believe it or not.

When winter comes, if you prepare correctly, you can continue your exercise routine both indoors and out. Here are a few tips to prevent your winter workout from becoming a chilling experience:

- Increase warm-up time by 5 to 10 minutes (preferably inside) even if you dance or march in place or go up and down the stairs.
- Drink 8 to 12 ounces of water before you leave and take along a bottle if you will be gone longer than 45 minutes to an hour. Sweat happens year round, not just in the summer!
- Stay warm and stay dry.

Bright Idea!

Freeze a paper cup filled with water. Next time your workout leaves you sore, peel back the paper on the cup and ice down that achy spot. Ice reduces swelling and pain. Don't forget the athletes' RICE formula: rest, ice, compression, and elevation, with the emphasis on ice. Once the swelling and pain have begun to subside, it's time to move the body part to prevent stiffness and atrophy (a reduction in the size) of the muscle.

Activities and Exercises to Keep You Young

Using the suggestions given below, find the exercises and activities you enjoy ... then do them. Choose activities that are pleasurable and that you will stick with—and don't forget, housework and gardening are excellent forms of exercise if you really put your body in motion. Depending on your personal fitness level, vary the exercises to keep from getting bored. Doing the same exercise repeatedly is like having a peanut butter and jelly sandwich every day for lunch—it just gets old.

Active play with children	Mopping floors
Aerobics (high or low impact)	Mowing the yard
Badminton	Rollerskating
Baseball	Rowing
Basketball	Running
Biking (both outdoors and indoors)	Soccer
Bowling	Softball
Dancing	Stair climbing
Gardening	Strength training
Golf	Swimming
Gymnastics	T'ai Chi
Handball	Tae Kwon Do

High-impact aerobics	Tennis
Hiking	Vacuuming
House cleaning	Volleyball
In-line skating	Walking
Karate	Washing windows
Kick boxing	Water exercises
Jumping rope	Yoga
Mall walking	

Tip 3: Make it a date. Put exercise activities for the week on your calendar along with other daily appointments. This designated time to exercise must be considered as important as family or work commitments or even time spent with community obligations. If your day flows according to your calendar and time for exercise is missing, you may see this as not important or another "unpleasant task" you will get to *if* time allows. Usually that "if" never happens! Making exercise a priority in your daily schedule is the only way it will ever become part of your life.

Tip 4: Take your own baseline measurements. While our focus is not on the scales or your weight, we do believe a baseline or starting point will let you see how exercise and activity can change your body for the better.

Using a tape measure, measure your waist, hips (at the widest area), and thighs (at the widest area). Also weigh in the buff in the morning and get someone to measure your height. Enter your height, weight, waist, hips, and thigh measurements in your personal training diary. Check your weight and other measurements every 2 to 4 weeks, and again record these measures in your diary.

Tip 5: Partner with a pal. J. Raglin, Ph.D., from the Indiana University Department of Kinesiology, found that spouses who worked out with their partners had a dropout rate of only 6.3

percent compared with spouses who worked out without their partners. This "single" group had an astounding 43 percent drop-out rate. Most researchers agree that you will realize the greatest long-term success with exercise if you have a spouse, loved one, or friend join you. A partner acts as your coach, motivator, and conscience, as well as someone to share your success and failure with. Choosing a reward that you can enjoy together can also help to keep you motivated with the EAT Plan.

Tip 6: Make sure you have proper clothing. This means having a base layer, a warmth layer, and a windproof layer.

- **Base layer:** Choose shirts and tights of a fabric that pulls sweat from the body. Blends such as Nike's Dri-fit and Dupont's Coolmax are reliable. Remember, cotton stays damp when wet with sweat, and dampness will make you even colder during icy weather!
- **Warmth layer:** Consider layering with more than one piece like a turtleneck and then zippered layer or pullover. That way you can pull off a layer as you warm up or if the temperature increases. When your body is cold, it sends more blood to the midsection to protect your vital organs at the expense of your head, feet and hands, so don't forget a hat or hood (since the body loses a lot of heat from the head) and gloves or mittens (mittens are better since they allow the fingers to keep each other warm). Socks should be polyester or wool just like your mittens.
- **Windproof layer:** Look for water-resistant, lightweight, and breathable items (both top and bottom, if it's raining).

Forget Going for the Burn

While you're getting your clothing together for the kickoff exercise day, don't forget sunscreen. This is not just for summer anymore, as you can get sunburned snow skiing or mountain climbing. Use a sunscreen with a sun protection factor (SPF) of at least 15, and be sure to apply it 30 minutes before you are ready to go so it can do its job properly.

Care for the Sole

Exercise shoes are now sport specific, and it might take some time to find the right fit at the right price. Be sure to try on your shoes with the type of socks that you will be wearing to exercise, and make sure your toes have plenty of room in the toe box. Walk around in the store for a few minutes to see if the shoes rub or are uncomfortable in any way. If they are pinching now, just think how they will feel in the midst of your run or basketball game.

Red Alert
Protect yourself from injury: If you are going out at night, wear a jacket with reflective material.

Tip 7: Fuel your fitness. Whether you work at home or an office, you have to make your snacks count to deactivate stress-aging and have enough energy to really *move* with exercise. If you've gotten caught up in the fad that if a food is labeled "low-fat" or "fat-free," you can eat the entire package, think again. The label "low-fat" or "fat-free" can often mean low-fiber, low-nutrition, and high-sugar. For many of us, our diet has become one of processed, packaged fat-free foods that rate a big nutritional zero when it comes to fiber or nutrient content.

Think M&Ms

Few of us sit down to three squares a day anymore. In that regard, now more than ever it's vital to think about what you choose to fuel your body. With the EAT Plan, we want you to think **mixed minimeals:** the dynamite duo. These minimeals that you graze on should be a combination of a lean protein source and a carbohydrate, such as a chicken wrap *(sans* sauce) or a bean burrito.

However, before you start spreading food on the counter celebrating your new freedom to snack, be aware that mixed minimeals are not a license to pig out. Keep your portions *small.* According to Thomas Wolever, M.D., associate professor at the University of Toronto Department of Nutritional Sciences, eating between nine and seventeen minimeals as opposed to three big meals can reduce total blood cholesterol and LDL cholesterol (the bad stuff) by about 8 to 12 percent.

Also, did you know your stomach is only about the size of a grapefruit when empty? Hard to believe? Well, keep reading. Investigators at Columbia University's Obesity Research Center found that people could hold about 4 cups of water in their stomach prior to dieting. Yet after losing from 12 to 28 pounds, they could hold less than 3 cups, or a decline of about 27 percent. Obesity per se doesn't increase stomach capacity, but overeating too many calories over the course of the day does. The problem with this stretching is that the stomach sends signals of fullness to the brain only when the stomach reaches a certain point of fullness. Therefore, the more your stomach can hold, the larger the meal needed to tell your brain that you have eaten enough.

The amazing good news is that when your stomach becomes used to smaller meals (which happens when you eat small, frequent mixed minimeals), the less food it takes to inform the brain that you are full.

Energy Zapper 1: Too much sugar can cause a rapid increase in blood sugar followed by a plunge that leaves you feeling exhausted. Combine a small amount of protein with your carbohydrate for energy over the long haul.

Energy Zapper 2: Too much caffeine can dehydrate you. Offset every caffeine product with 2 glasses of water.

Energy Zapper 3: When you skip breakfast and/or lunch, your body will feel like it never shifts out of neutral all day. This is like trying to run your car when the gas gauge is on empty.

Energy Zapper 4: When you drink very little water throughout the day, your energy level will fade as the day progresses.

Bodybuilding Bonus Foods

The following Circle of Ten Fitness Foods provide you with the energy nutrients needed (protein, fat, and carbohydrate) as well as fiber, vitamins, and minerals that work with your body and exercise plan to burn fat and build muscle. These foods are pulled from the lists in Deactivator 1. Along with drinking plenty of water each day, try to include three of these powerhouse energy foods each day:

Circle of Ten Fitness Foods

Water	For hydration of your body and skin
Whole grain crackers	For fiber and carbohydrate

Sweet potatoes	Good carbohydrate boost plus antioxidants
Beans/legumes	Low fat, good source of protein, carbohydrate, and iron
Tomatoes	Contains cancer-fighting lycopene and very versatile
Skim milk/ yogurt	Great source of calcium and protein
Oranges	Loaded with vitamin C, folic acid, and fiber
Lean red meat/ dark meat poultry	Great for iron and zinc, low in fat
Broccoli	Packed with vitamins A and C, rich in fiber and potassium
Banana	Easy to carry and eat, quick carbo source, loaded with potassium and about 70 percent water

Tip 8: Always have water or snacks nearby. The ACSM suggests that you drink 2 glasses (about 16 ounces) of water 2 hours *before* exercise. If drinking water is part of your daily routine already, this will be a piece of cake. If you are not used to drinking water throughout the day, start thinking of water as a natural elixir for your younger-looking body:

More water = better-looking skin
More water = less fatigue

During your workout, drink another cup (about 8 ounces) of water every 15 to 20 minutes. If you go for an hour or more, add 30 to 60 grams of carbohydrate, which is equal to 120 to 240 calories (4 calories per gram of carbohydrate). You need that additional energy as fuel for your body and brain and to maintain your blood sugar level. Try a sports drink, cereal bar, large banana, fig cookies, or grapes. A sports drink should have carbohydrate concentration of 6 to 8 percent or about 14 to 19 grams per 8 ounces.

Sometimes drinks with a higher concentration of carbs, such as orange juice or soda, will slow fluid absorption and cause stomach cramps unless diluted. Also, sodas tend to dehydrate the body rather than rehydrate. The electrolytes that sports drinks contain (mainly sodium and potassium) aid in rehydration by increasing fluid absorption by your body. Cool water or drinks will work to increase the speed of absorption.

Lastly, it's a good idea to weigh yourself before and after exercise, and drink 2 glasses of water for every pound you lose. Now we are not talking about fat loss. Rather, we are talking about water loss (dehydration) from your workout, which needs to be replaced so that your body is adequately hydrated. Even sitting outside in the heat watching your son's soccer game for 2 hours can require as much as 2 to 4 glasses of water, and the only thing that's getting an aerobic workout is probably your mouth! One hour of tennis can require from 2 to 10 extra 8-ounce glasses of water, depending on the level of play and the heat.

Ten Energy Activators

Got a hectic schedule? Snack on these ten energy activators for a quick energy burst:

Popcorn	Dried fruit mix
Toaster waffles	Grapes
Vegetable juice	Fig bars
Energy bars (when you are so pushed	Low-fat yogurt
you wouldn't eat otherwise)	Instant oatmeal
	Bagels

Tip 9: Motivate yourself with a reward system. In Step 2, you listed your personal goals. What about your reward for achieving your goals? It is kind of like getting a promotion or a raise for a job well done but this reward is something you give yourself. You could start small, such as a new water bottle after you have added activities to your schedule for 2 weeks; you can bump up to buying some much-needed walking shoes after you schedule and complete activities for a month. You decide what the reward will be and note it by the goal. Give yourself something to look forward to . . . makes it much more fun and motivating!

Tip 10: Go for it! Decide on a date to start and go for it! Remember that there are going to be good days and bad days . . . days you *don't* feel like getting up, much less exercising. There will be times when you have to miss a week or two, because of life's interruptions that just happen and throw you off course. You may miss several weeks during cold and flu season when you can barely crawl to work, much less run on your treadmill.

Forget beating yourself up over what appears as failure. It is just a temporary setback, and everyone faces them, even star athletes. The important thing is to get past it and *not give up or quit.* Think of your commitment to increased activity as a work in progress. It takes time. You must reevaluate your commitment and goals from time to time, then start over again. The more you start to look at your time for activity as equally important to your life (and youthful good looks and health) as all of the other components in the EAT Plan, it will become easier, more natural, and a total part of all you do.

Red Flag

If you do miss a couple of weeks, pick up at a pace a bit below where you left off so you can ease your body back into its new regimen.

Step 3: Create Your Personal Home Gym

If you'd rather exercise in the comfort of your home, you're not alone. Many people enjoy exercising in private. As one client, Caroline, said, "I can feel free to shake, sweat, and bounce without feeling like I'm being watched by anyone. Exercising at home lets me really move my buns and also work at my own pace."

There are all sorts of popular exercise videos for all levels of fitness that will allow you to "move your buns," as Caroline said, and do so in the privacy of your own home. The convenient part of exercising at home is that you just get up 10 minutes earlier, pop in the tape, and get moving—no matter how inclement the weather is outside. Yes, there are *no* excuses!

The good news is you don't have to break the bank or even join a gym to get a good workout at home as you can build your own—right in your den or on your porch. Check the classified advertisements for used exercise equipment such as electronic treadmills or stationary bicycles, but be sure to use them for more than hanging clothes on at the end of the day.

Other basics that are great for a home-based gym include:

Step bench: A plastic bench that comes with adjustable risers serves a dual purpose. You can use it as a weight bench or for aerobics. Make sure it is made of tough plastic and is adjustable for safe and effective height.

Rubber mats: Comfortable for doing floor exercises as well as protecting floors from dumbbells.

Dumbbells: More versatile than a weight machine, you'll need pairs of 3, 5, and 8 pounds if you are just starting and later add 10- and 12-pound pairs. If you are more experienced, check out a free-weight set but you will need a pal to spot for you as you use heavier weights.

Workout gloves: To protect hands from metal weight bars.

Exercise bands or tubes: Opt for three different colors that provide three different levels of resistance. You can work almost all muscle groups. Most sets come with instructional guides or demonstration videos.

Home fitness book: Check out your library or bookstore for easy-to-follow guides.

These exercise tools are optional, but also fun and useful:

Fit ball: After years of use by physical therapists, you can now get one for home. It's great for stretching your lower back and doing abdominal and leg work. These giant inflatable balls come in a variety of different sizes and colors. Sit down on it and make sure your thighs are parallel to the floor for a correct fit.

Heart-rate monitor: A little more pricey than the other items but it's a great reward for making your goal. Look for a wristwatch size that has a continuous readout of your heart rate. Use it to pace yourself and keep on track during aerobic workouts.

Mirrors: Important to see that your form is correct, but mirrors are also great motivation as you see those muscles becoming toned.

Just the Facts

Here's some delightful music to your ear (and rear)! Researchers in the Department of Physical Therapy at Springfield College in Massachusetts found that people who exercise to music will stay with it longer than if they work out in silence. Men and women riding stationary bikes rode from 25 to 29 percent longer listening to their favorite tunes.

Step 4: Putting It All Together

Now that you've gone through the first three steps of Age Deactivator 4, we're going to give you a revitalizing fitness plan to follow this week—and every week from now on. Look through the Revitalizing Weekly Fitness Checklist and check off each tip as you progress with your program.

Revitalizing Weekly Fitness Checklist

_____ Set goal for the week.
_____ Choose type of activities for the week.
          Walking or other aerobic activity (3 times a week)
          Weight training (at least 2 times a week)

Stretching (daily)
Activities such as gardening, walking the dog or playing
with the kids (daily)
____ Mark off "activity time" on your calendar to meet weekly
goal.
____ Partner with a pal.
____ Have necessary clothes/equipment ready.
____ Keep sunscreen handy.
____ Have snacks and water/sports drink ready, depending on
activity and time.
____ Continue eating your Circle of Ten foods daily.
____ Reward yourself for meeting your goal.

Sample Revitalizing Daily Fitness Plan

Monday

Goal: Walk for 25 to 30 minutes.
Activity: Walk dog for 10 minutes before work.
Walk with Sonja for 15 to 20 minutes during kids'
soccer practice.
Partner: Leave Sonja a message about walking during soccer
practice.
Equipment: Put walking shoes, socks, sunscreen, and visor in
gym bag.
Snacks/water: Put bottle water and dried fruit in gym bag.

It's Never Too Late

You did it, didn't you? The kids and the soccer ball aren't
the only ones moving around now as you've made time for
yourself to get back in shape. As you move into Age Deactivator
5, you will continue to set your weekly exercise goals, as you
have continued with Age Deactivators 1 to 3. If you have an

extra break in your day, don't go plop on the couch with the TV remote in hand. Instead, take advantage of this time to stretch, touch, reach, and bend as you get back in touch with the new youthful, flexible body you're working toward.

We all know that time triggers change. What may have worked for you yesterday as you swam laps in the pool or ran track with your college's cross-country team may not work for you today. But we know that you can embrace that million-dollar racehorse (or Mercedes-Benz!) and experience peak performance in all you do as you reassess your priorities, refresh your commitment to good health and activity, and take a new look at yourself—the younger you!

Let the EAT Plan continue to be your guide to vitality and youthful living as you turn the page and start Age Deactivator 5.

Age Deactivator 5

find Relief for a Hard Day's Night:

EAT to Sleep Well and Feel Rested

Sleep deprivation was written all across Kelly's face. Until she started the EAT Plan 2 years ago, this 45-year-old woman lived for months with dark circles under her eyes from lack of restful sleep. Kelly made it a point to be in bed by 9:00 P.M., but then she tossed and turned until sunrise and always felt almost too tired to go to work the next day, much less exercise or be active.

Like Kelly, many of our clients and seminar participants claim to be exhausted—all the time. One 40-year-old hospital administrator said, "I go to bed tired and feel tired all night. I awaken tired, then I feel tired the next day."

Shannon, a 31-year-old stay-at-home mom, complained, "No matter how much I sleep, it's never restful." She told of her sleep being interrupted by frequent awakening and becoming awake enough that she remembered these times the next day. Perhaps even more common are awakenings that clients have where they do not remember waking up but feel the result of a definite break in their "deep" sleep.

If getting good sleep is your problem, you're not alone. One third of the adult population reports sleep difficulties and one half of all menopausal women don't sleep well or long enough, according to the National Sleep Foundation. A March 1997 survey in *Consumer Reports* noted even greater sleep problems. Half of the men and two thirds of the women said they frequently had problems getting a good night's sleep. More than half of these had trouble sleeping at least 3 nights a week, and for 12 percent it was a daily problem.

Because obtaining restful sleep is mandatory for deactivating stress-aging, it is helpful to understand the characteristics of normal sleep and how any deviation from this will make you feel old and tired.

The Stages of Sleep

While it may seem that all sleep is the same throughout the night, you are actually undergoing various stages of sleep and each serves a unique function. For example, immediately upon falling asleep, you move from a light sleep to a deeper form of sleep. It is during deep sleep that you experience metabolic and tissue restoration. Growth hormone is also secreted, and stress hormones are at a minimum.

"No stress hormones? Maybe if I slept twenty-four hours a day, my blood pressure would be normal!" Not only did the recent downsizing of Gary's corporation leave him out of a job but his stress hormones were wreaking havoc with his body, causing his blood pressure to shoot up. This 51-year-old man desperately wanted answers as to how to stop stress-aging before more problems occurred. Keep listening, we told Gary, for sleep gets more complicated as you progress through the night.

After about 90 minutes of deep sleep, you move to REM (rapid eye movement) sleep. This is when you dream, and your body is more active. REM sleep restores your nervous system, processes information, and fixes memories. Then you shift gears again and drift back into deep sleep. These stages alternate throughout the night, with REM sleep increasing each period and deep sleep decreasing. To be fully renewed in the morning, you need ample amounts of each type of sleep.

Sleep problems occur at every age but generally become more frequent during middle age and are most prevalent in the elderly. Like we're telling you something new, right? Older adults actually need the same amount of sleep they did when they were young, but lighter sleep, medical problems, medications, and daytime naps can interfere with night sleep, making it shorter and more disrupted. The most serious problem of poor sleep is that it affects every part of your life—your disposition; your relationships; your ability to think, reason, and be creative; and your productivity. In addition, a study by Martica Hall, Ph.D., a postdoctoral fellow in the Department of Psychiatry at the University of Pittsburgh School of Medicine, reported that sleep disruptions weaken the immune system and therefore can activate stress-aging. This is certainly not something you want to happen.

Ben Franklin Couldn't Sleep Either

Thanks to Benjamin Franklin, electricity has enabled us to push back bedtime with artificial light and television for entertainment. (Ironically, Ben Franklin had chronic sleep problems, according to history books!) Before the invention of electric lights, the average American got 10 hours of sleep each night. Today, the average American gets only 7 hours of sleep.

When you finally do go to bed, your mind is alert with all of the things on your list for the next day. When you do awaken to a blaring alarm, you feel more exhausted than when you went to bed. You might be able to handle a few nights of poor sleep, yet over time, this sleep debt can increase, the cycle will continue, and it will show—in your looks, attitude, and alertness.

"Java. Just drink coffee—a lot of coffee—so you don't feel so tired." So that's how you resolve your poor sleeping habits? Yes, it is possible to carry a large sleep deficit and not feel sleepy as long as you stay stimulated or pumped up. Perhaps this explains the resurgence of coffeehouses with all the specialty blends, along with newly developed higher-caffeine soft drinks. Nonetheless, eventually this sleep debt will translate into symptoms of stress-aging, including moodiness, irritability, depression, reduced physical and mental performance, lessened ability to bounce back from stress, impaired immune function, and a tendency to be accident-prone.

Here's a word of caution to those who think little sleep and pots of coffee will average out. Don't drive too fast after a night of poor sleep. Many car crashes are due to inattention and fatigue, while industrial accidents are caused by faulty transfer of information. Remember the terrible oil spill of the Exxon *Valdez* that occurred because the first mate was asleep at the wheel and ignored warning signals?

There's a better way to keep stress-aging at bay than to sleep 24 hours a day, as Gary suggested. Using our eight steps in Age Deactivator 5, you will now learn some surefire tips on how to get to sleep, stay asleep, and awaken feeling rested as you benefit from the youth-boosting rejuvenation that occurs with sleep.

Step 1: Evaluate Foods That May Cause Lack of Sleep

Since we are nutritionists, and this is the EAT Plan, we believe that food is an important aspect in staying young. In that regard, some food can also activate stress-aging, especially if it is hindering restful sleep.

Let's see what you've been eating that can contribute to your lack of sleep. Most people don't think of food as a possible stimulant but it can be depending on its chemical composition.

Check off the following foods or medications you consume regularly.

_____ Coffee
_____ Soft drinks
_____ Tea
_____ Chocolate candy or dessert
_____ Chocolate milk, hot chocolate, or cocoa
_____ Jalapeño peppers
_____ Onions
_____ Alcohol (wine, beer, or liquor)
_____ Rich desserts
_____ Rich sauces
_____ Tobacco
_____ Medications such as prescription diet pills (amphetamines), antidepressants, asthma medications, cold preparations with pseudoephredrine, nasal decongestants, pain relievers containing caffeine, thyroid hormone, some drugs for high blood pressure, steroids, and sleeping pills

All these foods or medications can greatly interfere with your good night's sleep. The more you consume, and the closer to bedtime, the greater the chance that you'll be up counting sheep—certainly not something you want to do if looking and feeling younger is important! Try to limit your intake of these foods especially during the late afternoon or evening.

Step 2: Determine Your Sleep Readiness

Now that you see where your pitfalls are with foods and medications, we want you to evaluate your sleep readiness. Just as we all prefer different foods or even have different eating styles, we also differ in our sleeping habits.

Go through our list of sleep steps and find out what type of sleeper you are, then we will help you improve your chance for a restful night.

Steps to Good Sleep

Work through the sleep steps for about 14 nights to determine what type of sleeper you are.

1. On a day when you don't have to get up at a certain time, we want you to try to measure how long you would naturally sleep *if* you go to bed at your regular time. Now this step works best on a weekend with no alarm or noises to wake you up artificially. Ideally, you should awaken naturally feeling refreshed, healthy, and energetic the next morning.
2. After you have tested yourself at least 5 times, take the average number of hours you slept as your ideal number. This number varies greatly but the average number of hours needed by most adults is still 8 to 9 hours per night.
3. If you wake up during the night, keep a record each time of how long you're awake, at what time, and what you do while you are awake.
4. If you wake up and worry, keep a list by your bed to write down your worries as they occur.
5. Count the number of episodes of awakening each night for at least the next 2 weeks.

Once you've gone through the above five steps, we want you to check out the following list of sleep types, along with suggestions for how to accommodate the specific type and still get the sleep you need.

Light Sleeper

Problem: I fall asleep easily but every little noise wakes me up.

Solution: Use barriers such as ear plugs or a night mask to keep distractions at bay.

Can't Fall Asleep Sleeper

Problem: I take a long time to fall asleep but sleep well once asleep.

Solution: Dose yourself with light for an hour or two each morning to reset your biological clock.

Up and Down Sleeper

Problem: I awaken frequently during the night but fall right back to sleep after each time.

Solution: Could be a symptom of diabetes if frequent urination is the cause. See your physician to rule out physical causes.

Early to Bed, Early to Rise Sleeper

Problem: I fall asleep early but then I awaken too early and cannot get back to sleep.

Solution: A walk before dark may help to reset your biological clock.

Night Owl Sleeper

Problem: I cannot go to sleep before midnight and prefer to sleep until mid- to late morning or afternoon.

Solution: Unless your daytime schedule keeps you from sleeping late, you are probably getting enough sleep.

Early Bird Sleeper

Problem: I fall asleep early (9:00 to 10:00 P.M.) but awaken early (5:00 to 6:00 A.M.).

Solution: As long as your schedule permits you to go to bed early, you are probably getting ample sleep to deactivate stress-aging.

Day Sleeper

Problem: I nod off frequently during the day.

Solution: You may be sleep deficient due to a sleep disorder. Daytime sleepiness is one of the key symptoms of snoring or obstructive sleep apnea. Try to increase sleep time at night, or see your doctor for an evaluation.

Step 3: EAT to Improve Your Snooze

Rare is the person who can climb into bed at night without a little bedtime snack. While that glass of warm milk your mother brought to you as a child can help you fall asleep, the only reason is that it's soothing for someone you love (like Mom!) to fix you a warm glass of milk. Chemically, it's carbohydrate that has a calming, drowsiness-inducing effect, not protein, like that in milk.

If sleep problems are making you feel old, choose from our list of Bedtime Snacks to improve your snooze.

Ten E-zzzy Bedtime Snacks

1. Pretzels
2. Cereal
3. Graham crackers

4. Fresh fruit
5. Dried fruit
6. Fruit juice
7. Vanilla wafers
8. Saltines or other low-fat crackers
9. Popcorn
10. Toast or bread with jam or jelly

Red Flag

Beware of drugs than can cause insomnia, including:

- Blood pressure drugs including some beta-blockers, clonidine, methyldopa, and reserpine
- Hormones, such as oral contraceptives, progesterone, thyroid drugs, or cortisone
- Bronchodilators and theophylline
- Anticancer drugs
- Phenytoin
- Levodopa
- Quinidine
- Nicotine
- Decongestants
- Over-the-counter pain and cold relievers containing caffeine (such as Anacin, Exedrin, and Empirin)

Before you reach over the counter for popular sleep aids, be sure to read this:

- Excedrin P.M., Nytol, and Benadryl all use an antihistamine to induce sleep. If you use any of these frequently, you will likely develop a tolerance.
- Melatonin is a natural hormone secreted by the pineal gland in the brain. As a general rule, production tends to decrease after age 40. Studies on the use of melatonin to promote sleep are inconclusive. As of now, there is no

consensus on either the effectiveness of melatonin or its safety. When it does help, REM sleep is increased by about one hour per night, deep sleep does not change. There is no data on the long-term side effects of taking melatonin, but be sure and watch for side effects including vivid and disturbing dreams, aggravated depression, and grogginess the morning after. If you do try it, take 1 to 3 milligrams if you are less than 40 years old, 2 to 6 milligrams if you are age 40 or older, 30 to 60 minutes before bedtime. A word of caution: Do not take melatonin if you are trying to get pregnant, are already pregnant, or have an autoimmune disease. Product purity is also an issue, and synthetic melatonin may be better than the natural hormone from animal sources because the dosages are more standardized.

Bright Idea!

To increase your melatonin level naturally, try these practices that promote natural melatonin:

- Make sure you are exposed to natural sunlight in the morning.
- If you go to work in the dark, take a walk when the sun is out to reset your internal clock.
- Take a hot bath or shower about two to three hours before bedtime.
- Make sure your bedroom is dark or use eye covers to sleep.
- Eat a high-carbohydrate snack from our Ten E-zzzy Bedtime Snacks List (pages 208–09).

- Valerian root, a popular herb, has been shown to reduce the time needed to fall asleep and to improve sleep quality. No morning grogginess has been reported. There is also no drug interaction with alcohol and no reports of addiction. One in ten people reports a stimulating effect instead of a sedating effect (including Deb, the creative writer for this book!). If you take valerian root, take it 30 to 45 minutes before bedtime as follows:

1 to 2 grams of the root as tea
1 to 1.5 teaspoons of tincture
150 to 300 milligrams of standardized valeric acid (the active ingredient)

- Chamomile is another popular sleepy time herb. There are two varieties, and both are useful. German chamomile is best used as a tea, while Roman chamomile has a bitter taste more appropriate as a tincture. Both types are calming and soothing before bed.
- Catnip is a stimulant for cats; however, in people it appears to work as a sedative similar to valerian. Drink catnip tea prepared from 1 to 2 teaspoons of the herb per cup.
- Passionflower has been found to produce prolonged sleeping time—in rats, that is. This common herb is widely used as a sedative in Great Britain, and like catnip and chamomile, it is generally used as a tea before bedtime.
- Hops is yet another herb that has been promoted recently as a sleep aid, but researchers have reported questionable beneficial effects.

Prescription Sleeping Medications

If your sleep problem is serious and you've discussed this with your physician, chances are you have inquired about sleeping pills. Keep in mind that sleeping pills are only appropriate when insomnia is acute or when it is extremely important to get a good night's sleep. While valium is the most frequently prescribed sleep aid, others include:

Restoril
Prosom
Doral
Dalmane
Halcion and Ambien (both are linked with temporary amnesia
as a side effect)

Bright Idea!
Don't forget the following Good Sleep Scents!
Orange blossom, marjoram, chamomile, and lavender have all
been connected to improved sleep when used as aromatherapy.
For more information on how to use these sleep scents, see Age
Deactivator 2.

Step 4: Change Your Attitude Toward Sleep

Ever tried so hard to sleep that you were more awake than
normal? Remember this: If you can't fall asleep within 20 minutes,
get up, and do something relaxing like reading, watching television (not enough to get interested; try low volume and a boring
station), taking a warm bath, listening to music, making love, or
relaxation techniques like meditation, visualization, or prayer.

How do other people fall asleep? A survey published in *USA
Today* (March 16, 1998) reported the following favorite remedies:

Reading	66%
TV	63%
Walk/exercise	47%
Pray/meditate	46%
Music/radio	44%
Bath/shower	43%
Limit caffeine	39%
Eat	24%
Take sleep aid	16%
Warm milk	10%

Check the Thermostat

The temperature of the room has a lot to do with how well we sleep. If unsure about your sleep "comfort zone," try a room temperature of between 65 and 70 degrees. The human body likes a cool but not cold temperature to sleep.

Just the Facts
Body temperature starts to drop around midnight, hitting its coldest point around 4:00 to 6:00 A.M., which is why many people wake up feeling chilled or with all the covers on. Body temperature then starts to rise and remains high throughout the rest of the day, which is why almost no one can sleep more than 2 or 3 hours during the daytime, even after being up all night and if the room is dark.

Step 5: Look Toward the Light

If you have trouble sleeping during a full moon, you can quit your howling. It may not be that odd after all, as light has intriguing effects on the human mind and body. It is well documented that light entering the eyes influences the pituitary and pineal glands, which control the entire endocrine system. At night, when it is dark, the brain produces less serotonin and more melatonin (the hormone naturally produced in the brain that helps us to sleep deeply). In fact, light therapy, using natural or artificial light, can cause physiological changes in the human body.

In light therapy, a special kind of light called broad-spectrum light is used to simulate the effect of having a few extra hours of daylight each day. People exposed to this bright light, using specially made "light boxes," subsequently produce serotonin, the neurotransmitter in the brain that has a calming, anxiety-reducing effect.

Because of this boost of serotonin, light therapy may ease

depression, which in many cases produces sleep disorders (whether too much sleep or an inability to maintain sleep).

Although for centuries people have used sunlight for healing, light therapy is a recent alternative treatment. At many medical schools, scientists are using bright light therapy to relieve the symptoms associated with seasonal affective disorder (SAD), a psychological problem that occurs with the change of seasons and less daytime exposure to light. Those who have SAD feel depressed and fatigued, and may crave carbohydrates, as these carbohydrates boost levels of serotonin in the body.

Light therapy is thought to be helpful for many physical and emotional problems, in addition to SAD, that involve changes in serotonin levels and circadian rhythm including: PMS, some types of migraine headaches, stress, and of course, insomnia.

If your sleep problems are overwhelming, ask your doctor about light therapy. Perhaps this natural way of resetting your body's clock can put the problem *and* your body to rest!

Just the Facts

In light therapy studies on women, participants with PMS reported less depression, less moodiness, better sleep, and better concentration. Researchers have shown that serotonin levels drop just before ovulation, and this drop correlates with the onset of PMS symptoms; serotonin levels rebound with the onset of menstruation or when PMS symptoms decrease. Recent research suggests that PMS occurs in women with low base levels of serotonin; when serotonin levels drop further at ovulation, these levels fall low enough for symptoms to appear. Using phototherapy, women with PMS can keep their serotonin-melatonin levels high enough to prevent their PMS symptoms from appearing.

Step 6: Use Mental Aerobics to Destress Before Slumber

We know you are ready to doze after all this soothing information on better sleep, but perk up for a few more minutes. There is still one more key area we need to share with you. Relaxation therapies can help you reduce stress so you get to sleep quickly and also fall back asleep in less time if you awaken during the night.

Using the Mind-Body Activities listed on pages 215 to 221, we want you to select the therapies that you will regularly use and practice them during the daytime. As you become efficient at doing these mental aerobics, your body will learn how to automatically switch from the pumping "fight or flight" response into a calmer, more peaceful mood. Studies show that when you withdraw from problems and use mind-body tools for relaxation, you can produce alpha and theta waves consistent with serenity and happiness and prepare your body for restful slumber.

Let's look at some of the most common forms of mind-body aerobics:

Autogenics. This method of "cuing" yourself to calm down and relax is easy to perform and can be done anywhere. Because the brain needs only a few reminders to calm down, autogenics teaches you to concentrate on raising the temperature of your hands and feet, since cold hands and feet are a symptom of stress. Proponents claim that autogenics will give your heart a break from pumping so hard, open blood vessels, reduce breathing rate and pulse, and lower blood pressure.

Sit quietly, and put your left hand in your lap, palm up. Lay your right palm on top of it, and clasp your fingers together. Concentrating on the feeling in your hands, "mindfully" work to raise the temperature of your hands for 10 minutes, then do the same with your feet. Counselors claim, if this is done correctly, you will feel the "heat" rise in your hands and feet.

Autogenics may be performed prior to bedtime to help put your body in a more peaceful mode conducive for sleep.

Deep Abdominal Breathing. Many people breathe from their chest, taking shallow, rapid breaths, but this type of breathing only hinders relaxation—and you have to relax to enjoy good sleep!

Taking slow, deep "abdominal" breaths not only oxygenates the brain, but helps to end the stress cycle and enables your heart rate and blood pressure to return to normal. The brain makes its own morphine-like pain relievers, called endorphins and enkephalins, that are associated with a happy, positive feeling and help relay "stop pain" messages. During deep abdominal breathing, you add oxygen to the blood and cause your body to release endorphins, while decreasing the release of stress hormones. How can you do this? Follow these easy steps:

1. Lie on your back in a quiet room with no distractions.
2. Place your hands on your abdomen, and take in a slow, deliberate deep breath through your nostrils. If your hands are rising and your abdomen is expanding, then you are breathing correctly. If your hands do not rise, yet you see your chest rising, you are breathing incorrectly.
3. Inhale to a count of 5, pause for 3 seconds, then exhale to a count of 5. Start with 10 repetitions of this exercise, then increase to 25, twice daily.

Guided Imagery or Visualization. Visualization (or guided imagery) is a stress-release activity that you can do wherever you are, any time of the day or night. If you awaken at 3:00 A.M., and find yourself too preoccupied to fall asleep, use visualization to put your mind at ease. This is a technique of focusing on your senses to create a desired state of relaxation in your mind. Take the following steps:

1. Find a place where you can be comfortable, allow about 15 minutes for this exercise. Take several deep breaths while sitting or lying down, and close your eyes.
2. Imagine a relaxing place—somewhere you have been before, so it can be visualized in your mind—such as the seashore at sunset or sunrise, a mountain cabin next to a babbling brook, or a raft on a lake on a sunny day.
3. Continue to breathe slowly and keep this image in your mind. As you explore your mental picture of your relaxing spot, imagine all the stress, worries, and tension leaving your body. Feel the temperature of your special place. See the colors surrounding you. What sounds do you hear? Smell the freshness of the air. Touch the gentleness of the moment. Take in all the sensory details of your relaxing place and continue to destress.
4. After about 15 minutes, slowly open your eyes and acclimate yourself to the surroundings in the room. Stretch your arms and legs; gently move your head from side to side and feel the tension release. Carry the calm feeling you now have with you through the day.

If you have trouble imagining scenes and images, recordings of waves or rain can help. Or purchase postcards with peaceful, serene scenes on them, and keep these with you. Pull out your visualization cards when you feel your body tensing and you need to imagine being somewhere else where life is kinder and less threatening.

Laughter Therapy. Can a laugh a day help you to sleep soundly? Maybe, according to some researchers. The average adult laughs only about 17 times a day, while a 6-year-old laughs as many as 300 times. Yet laughter helps to relieve anxiety, decreases stress-producing hormones, and increases immune system activity. Laughter may even have an aerobic benefit. Dr. William F. Fry, a psychiatrist at the Stanford University School of Medicine, has studied the aerobic, physical, and emotional benefits that laughter can give and found that 100 laughs are equivalent to 10 minutes spent rowing.

Now, if you spent time "rowing" each day, wouldn't you sleep like a baby? Well, if you are not near a lake or river and have no access to a shell for rowing practice, we advise you to start chuckling more. It's free. It's fun. And your healing sleep may depend on it.

Meditation. Remember when transcendental meditation (page 43) was considered a little wacky? Today many types of meditation are recognized as a viable way to lower blood pressure, reduce chronic pain, and more importantly to our current discussion, *alleviate insomnia.* This stress releaser seeks to integrate the mind, body, and spirit through the silent repetition of a focus word ("love"), sound ("om"), phrase ("peace heals"), or prayer ("thank you, God"). As thoughts intrude, you will continue to chant mindfully while facilitating the relaxation response. This technique can guide you beyond the negative thoughts and agitations of the busy mind and allow you to become "unstuck" from your worries and other disturbing emotions. Mindfulness is a traditional Buddhist approach to meditation and allows your mind to be full of whatever you are doing at that moment, whether dancing, gardening, writing, or listening to music. Intense focus is the key to mindfulness, which keeps negative thoughts from intruding on the moment.

Red Alert!
Some people who meditate only occasionally experience increased anxiety or fear rather than calm. Researchers believe that these feelings may be responses to the unfamiliar sensation of being totally relaxed and uninhibited.

Music Therapy. You can thank Pythagoras, the sixth-century B.C. philosopher and mathematician, for discovering this mind-body treatment. Music therapy is the use of music as an adjunctive therapy for treating neurological, mental, or behavioral disorders such as developmental and learning disabilities, Alzheimer's disease and other aging-related problems, brain injuries, autism, poor motor control, and acute and chronic pain. Today, there are more than 5,000 music therapists in the United States and Canada who use music to soothe and heal physiological and psychological problems. And studies are revealing that Mozart boosts intelligence. Ground-breaking research done at the University of California found that Mozart's "Sonata in D Major for Two Pianos" temporarily boosted students' abilities to distinguish shapes and objects—a higher-brain activity. Even surgeons report performing better when they are able to select the music played in the operating room.

The good news for those who have difficulty sleeping because their active mind is running in high gear, according to composer and researcher Steven Halpern, is that classical music can transport the listener's brain into the alpha state, a state of relaxation much like meditation. So try popping in that Vivaldi CD, lie down on your bed, and zone out while your body prepares for a good night's slumber.

Prayer. Prayer also allows your thoughts to take a break from daily analytical routines and gives support to the spiritual dimension of life. When you pray or meditate, your body switches from the pumping "fight or flight" response into a calmer, more peaceful mood. Like other forms of mental aerobics, both prayer and meditation have been proven to produce alpha and theta waves consistent with serenity and happiness.

Can prayer or meditation help you to fall asleep or stay asleep? Both help to relax the body and comfort the mind—two key factors needed for restful sleep.

Progressive Muscle Relaxation. Also known as deep muscle relaxation, this mind-body exercise involves the contraction and relaxation of all of the major muscle groups in the body. Beginning with the head and progressing to the neck, arms, hands, chest, back, stomach, pelvis, legs, and feet, tense each muscle group to the count of 10, then release to the count of 10. At the same time, it is important to perform deep abdominal breathing, breathing in while tensing the muscles, and breathing out or exhaling while relaxing them. You can do this exercise before going to bed or when you awaken in the middle of the night.

Relaxation Response. The relaxation response was first described by Dr. Herbert Benson more than 20 years ago. Benson realized that the ability to induce the relaxation response at will offered the potential to reduce physical strain and negative thoughts—and increase your ability to self-manage stress. Achieving relaxation through the relaxation response is important in helping you reduce the emotional stress of daily living. This is done by concentrating on breathing and developing an inner quiet and peacefulness, a calming of negative thoughts and worries, and a mental focus away from any problems.

And of course, relaxation increases your ability to fall alseep in less time. How can you learn the relaxation response? Try these easy steps:

1. Set aside a period of about 20 minutes that you can devote to relaxation practice.
2. Remove outside distractions that can disrupt your concentration: turn off the radio, the television, even the ringer on the telephone, if need be.
3. Lie flat on a bed or floor, or recline comfortably so that your whole body is supported, relieving as much tension or tightness in your muscles as you can. You can use a pillow or cushion under your head if this helps.
4. In your own way, try to imagine that every muscle in your body is now becoming loose, relaxed, and free of any excess tension. Picture all of the muscles in your body beginning to unwind; imagine them beginning to go loose and limp.
5. Concentrate on making your breathing even. As you exhale, picture your muscles becoming even more relaxed, as if you somehow breathe the tension away.
6. During the 20-minute period, remain as still as possible; try to focus your thoughts as much as possible on the immediate moment, and eliminate any outside thoughts that may compete for your attention.
7. At the end of 20 minutes, take a few moments to study and focus on the feelings and sensations you have achieved. Notice whether areas that felt tight and tense at first now feel looser and more relaxed, and whether any areas of tension or tightness remain. As you continue to practice the relaxation response, you will feel increasingly more relaxed and less tight or tense.

Step 7: Create Your Circle of Ten Sleep Inducers

To get sounder sleep, you will probably need to use a combination of steps, including exercise, the right foods, destressing strategies, and maybe even herbal tea, if needed. We want you now to create your own Circle of Ten Sleep Inducers. Because every-one has a different sleep concern, each person's list will be unique. Check out the following to get an idea of what to include in your list.

1. **Get regular exercise.** The sedentary lifestyle to which many have grown accustomed can leave you feeling rest-less and not tired. Aerobic exercise and weight training will help you fall asleep easier and more deeply. The best time to exercise for sounder sleep is late afternoon or 4 to 6 hours before bedtime. If possible, try to exercise outside to gain the extra benefit of natural sunlight. This will help set your body's circadian rhythm and allow regular sleep.

2. **Go light at night.** Eating large, high-fat meals in the evening can interfere with sleep because of prolonged digestion time.

3. **Eliminate stimulants, alcohol, and tobacco** at least 6 hours before bedtime.

4. **Check your medications.** Among the drugs that can keep you awake are prescription diet pills (like amphetamines), antidepressants, asthma meds, cold preparations with pseudoephredrine, nasal decongestants, pain relievers containing caffeine, thyroid hormone, some drugs for high blood pressure, and steroids. Ironically, even sleeping pills can keep you wide awake all night. Make sure you ask your doctor or pharmacist about your medications to see if they are impeding your ability to sleep soundly.

5. **Nap with caution.** While it's true that an occasional nap may help if you need a boost during the afternoon, especially if nighttime sleep has been limited, napping can also interfere with the next night's sleep. If you feel drowsy, try exercise instead of a nap. If you choose to

nap, limit it to no more than 30 minutes and before 3:00 P.M.

6. **Wait until you are truly sleepy to lie down.** If you are a light sleeper, spend less time in bed to get deeper, more efficient sleep. If you awaken at night, do something relaxing. Don't toss and turn if you are still awake after a reasonable time. Lying in bed awake does not cement the psychological connection between bed and sleep.

7. **Establish a routine.** Try to wake up at the same time every day regardless of when you fall asleep.

8. **Set aside a worry time.** You might make a time earlier in the day to worry and make lists. If you wake up at night, make sure you have a pen and paper so you can write your thoughts down. Then promise yourself you will deal with them the next day.

9. **Wind down with pleasant rituals.** If you always do the same thing before bed, it sets up a natural expectation that sleep will follow. What do people do before bedtime to unwind? You can read, talk, lie quietly listening to music, take a bath or shower, or practice meditation, prayer, or other relaxation techniques. Rituals are important for the psychological connections they create.

10. **Create an atmosphere conducive to sleep.** Keep your bedroom dark, quiet, well ventilated, and cool. In other words, your bedroom should be a haven away from worries, arguments, or work. Use ear plugs or a night mask to keep out light and other distracters.

Gentlemen, Start Your Engines:

EAT to Balance Hormones and Feel Young

"It started as a typical mother-daughter argument over how short to hem a skirt for school. I feel that at age sixteen, a macro miniskirt is inappropriate. Kristin yelled that all the girls wear short skirts and I was ruining her life." Thirty-nine-year-old Connie grimaced as she spoke about the "war zone" in her home, raising a hormonal teenager while experiencing the mood swings associated with perimenopause.

"I ran to my room crying," she continued, "and she ripped off the skirt, tossed it in the garbage, and stomped out the back door with tears streaming down her face."

Hormone havoc is nothing new for teenagers. But if you thought you were through with their characteristic effects at puberty, think again. Particularly in midlife, hormonal changes affect everything from your sleep, weight, and skin to your hair and mood—yes, mood. And no one needs to tell you that if you "aren't in the mood," this greatly affects your relationships, and not just sexual ones.

You are almost through with the EAT Plan. By now you should be feeling younger and more energetic as you deactivate stress-aging with Age Deactivators 1–5. This last step, Age Deactivator 6, will show both men and women how to tame those raging hormones with food.

Tearful for No Reason?

"I feel empty and apathetic," Mary Jane, age 49, shared at a recent seminar. "I go to lunch with my friends, and they are laughing and talking about their lives, but I can't get excited. It's as if someone pulled out my happiness plug, and I can't find how to plug it in again."

Mary Jane went on to tell about her new career as the owner of an upscale boutique in the historic district of her town and how her son just finished medical school. "I have so much to be excited about, but I can't get that happy feeling inside like I used to have."

If you identify with what Mary Jane is feeling, perhaps research performed by P. Bjorntorp with the Department of Heart and Lung Diseases at Sahlgren's Hospital, University of Göteborg, Sweden, will help you understand the reason Bjorntorp suggests that changes in cortisol (a stress hormone described on page xviii) secretion and decreased levels of sex steroids and growth hormone result in a cluster of symptoms such as low energy and perceived unhappiness, altered body composition, heart disease, and non-insulin-dependent diabetes. He refers to these as "premature aging processes." As you know, we call this *stress-aging*. Bjorntorp also suggests that psychosocial stressors, such as moving, losing a job, or losing a mate through divorce or death, as well as alcohol and smoking, are involved in "premature aging" (or stress-aging).

Endocrinologist Matthew Hardy at the Population Council has also performed research in the area of stress-aging and reports that stress causes a man's sperm count to decrease. Hardy discovered that stress hormones override the enzymes which help cells produce testosterone (necessary for sperm formation) and have a strong negative effect on the male reproductive system.

Menopause—No Longer Just a "Woman-Thing"

"Male menopause? No way! That's a woman-thing." Rick was the "macho" type who took pride in his muscular build. At age fifty-three, he could easily pass for someone fifteen years his junior. Spending many nights at the gym working out kept Rick in top shape, and he even competed in bodybuilding contests around the state. But as we told Rick, male menopause *is* a man-thing, and it's very real. In fact, with his symptoms of impotence and fatigue, he may be going through this life stage right now.

Male menopause, which some researchers call "andropause" or "viropause," refers to the loss of virility usually occurring during the forties and fifties when a man's strength, sex drive, and peace of mind all take a nose dive. Some men become depressed thinking that their best years are over. Others may make drastic changes like buying a sports car or having an affair. Like PMS, many say this "midlife crisis" is all in one's "head," but there are bona fide biological explanations for what's going on.

According to researchers at Bristol Urological Institute at Southmead Hospital in the United Kingdom, stress is a major factor in the various symptoms of male menopause, including fatigue. Another study conducted by scientists in the Department of Psychiatry at Geneva University Hospital in Switzerland, found that the stress hormone, cortisol, increased in men during anticipatory stress while the levels of total testosterone and LH (luteinizing hormone) decreased. The greater the stress level and production of stress hormones, the more negative the effect on male menopausal symptoms.

Stress also negatively affects both men's and women's interest in sex. A man's sex drive is steered by testosterone, which as we just saw decreases in response to stress. A woman's sexual interest is more driven by her peace of mind and surrounding environment, and rises when she feels healthy, relaxed, contented, and financially secure. Now the EAT Plan cannot help you feel financially secure, but it can help you achieve improved health, greater relaxation, and ongoing contentment—all necessary for increasing that sex drive again! (And when you think about it, with better health and reduced stress, you may have more energy and productivity, leading to financial gain.)

The Signs of Male Menopause

"So what do I have to look forward to? Am I going to have hot flashes like my wife? Are we both going to be crabby all the time?" We honestly felt as if we were taking part of Rick's life away as we explained the reality of aging for men—something most men know *nothing* about. Besides depression, men may also experience the following:

Anxiety
Irritability
Decrease in energy
Erectile dysfunction
Loss of interest in sex
Weight gain
Sleeplessness
Delayed healing

Whether these symptoms qualify as menopause or not is debatable, but the changes to a man are real and affect his quality of life much as menopause does a woman's. Just like estrogen benefits women, a little testosterone can make a big difference in some men.

We praised Rick for continuing to work out to keep his body muscular. This will give him greater protection as he ages, for men's bodies do change. For example, between the ages of 40 and 70, a man loses 12 to 20 pounds of muscle, 15 percent of his bone mass, and 2 inches in height. If that isn't enough of a loss, consider these stats: A man's body metabolism also slows down, and after the age of 40, his testicles shrink slightly and sperm production declines. In addition, connective tissue in the prostate gland thickens, leading to problems with urination and ejaculation. The functioning of the penis becomes sluggish as the chambers responsible for erection fill with connective tissue and its supporting arteries narrow. While the testosterone loss is subtle compared to the estrogen decline in women, the levels do drop about 1 percent per year after age 40, resulting in a 30 percent decline by age 70. Believe it or not, some men experience severe enough drops in their testosterone levels that they have the hot flashes and night sweats associated with menopause.

Red Flag

If you think only women get osteoporosis or thinning of the bones, think again. Twenty-five percent of osteoporosis and fractures happen in men, including hip and spine fractures. The main risk factor for men is *age*. While men do not have a sudden decline in bone mass at middle age the way postmenopausal women do, their more subtle losses add up. In fact, the longer a man lives, the greater his chances are of suffering a fracture due to osteoporosis. After age 80, *one in four men* will suffer a broken hip, and *one in seven* will have a spinal fracture sometime in their lives.

''Well, do I need to get some hormone replacement therapy like my wife?'' Rick kept his voice low, trying to hide his nervousness about this new idea of male menopause. As we told Rick, this is a question scientists are still debating. Testosterone revs up the engine of sexual desire in both sexes and is also responsible for a man's secondary sexual characteristics including the beard, muscles, thick skin, and, possibly an aggressive attitude at work. On the other hand, Georgia State researcher James Dabbs, Ph.D., found that men with high testosterone levels responded negatively to the frustrations and challenges of a stressful job.

At this time, most researchers believe that the negative risks of taking testosterone supplements may outweigh the benefits. On one hand, testosterone supplements may reduce the effects of aging. However, on the negative side, too much testosterone can cause sterility in men, and even small amounts may contribute to tumor development. Testosterone also increases the production of red blood cells, thickening the blood and possibly increasing the risk of stroke.

Step 1: Know Your Testosterone Number

Who doesn't know their blood pressure reading? And surely you know what your cholesterol is. But if you are a male, do you know what your testosterone number is? Especially if you are age 40 and above, or if you are having symptoms that might be related to low testosterone, having this level checked by your health care provider may be a giant step toward reclaiming your youth. This baseline level can also be used to compare against future measurements.

Men function well at testosterone levels from *200 to 1,000* nanograms/milliliter (ng/ml), so it is often difficult to pinpoint a specific "low level." If you experience symptoms that concern you and your testosterone level proves to be in the low range, then hormone supplementation may be suggested by your physician.

Weighing the Benefits of Testosterone Supplements

Benefits	Risks	Costs
Maintains energy, libido, and muscle mass; reduces total cholesterol.	Reduces HDL cholesterol, blocks sperm production, and possibly stimulates prostate tumors	$50 to $100 a month by injection, pill, or patch

Step 2: Be Discerning with the New "Miracle" Aging Cures

From Rogaine to ab rollers to herbal concoctions, how you look and perform are big business. Some men are turning to hormone supplements such as DHEA, melatonin, and growth hormone. Often referred to as the superhormones, these big three make promises to slow or reverse the aging process. But is this always the smartest move? Maybe not, as the studies are still not complete. At this time the National Institute on Aging (NIA) is in the midst of a program to evaluate hormone therapy as a way to improve quality of life for the elderly.

"They're still studying whether this will work? I want it now, not when I'm an old man." Remember Rick? He was the first to ask where he could purchase growth hormone to keep his brawny physique the rest of his life.

Sure, we all want it now! Between the media hype and the "wonder drug" books, over $325 million dollars a year are spent on DHEA and melatonin combined. Yet in the midst of wanting to turn back time, very few reputable scientific studies have been conducted that show the long-term effects of these "miracle" supplements. Our advice?

- Be discerning.
- Check the facts.
- Talk with your doctor.

Never take a "miracle" cure unless you have thoroughly read the literature and discussed it with your doctor. Most of the time, if it sounds too good to be true, it is!

Lingo Lowdown

Hormones are chemical powerhouses that control a host of functions including growth, metabolism, digestion, sexual development, and reproduction. Too much or too little can lead to problems such as diabetes and weak bones.

Weighing the Benefits of DHEA Supplements

Both men and women produce dehydroepiandrosterone (DHEA) in their adrenal glands, and men at a slightly higher level. It floods the body during youth, then dwindles as we age. DHEA also aids in the production of sex hormones, particularly testosterone and estrogen, and may have a possible role in treating lupus. The jury is still out on whether DHEA is safe to take but stay on the alert as new studies are due out soon.

Touted Benefits	Known Risks	Cost
Increases energy and libido; improves mood; preserves muscle; strengthens immune system; and prevents cancer and heart disease.	Untested in human long-term clinical trials for safety and dosage strength; purity unregulated; may speed of up growth of prostate and endometrial cancer.	$5–$10 a month; over the counter.

Weighing the Benefits of Pregnenolone Supplements

Pregnenolone, a sex hormone precursor (to DHEA), often is referred to as the mother steroid hormone.

Touted Benefits	Known Risks	Cost
Strengthens skin; prevents wrinkles.	Little is known about long-term effects; overall risk factors uncertain.	$3.50–$7.00 a month; over the counter.

Weighing the Benefits of Melatonin Supplements

Melatonin is yet another popular hormone that can be purchased at any drug or natural food store. It is produced in the pea-size pineal gland in the center of the brain, and regulates the body's circadium rhythms (daily rhythms such as your sleep-wake cycle).

Touted Benefits	Known Risks	Cost
Improved sleep; boosts immunity; prevents cancer by protecting cells from free radicals.	Unregulated and untested for long-term; may cause depression and grogginess; not safe if you have immune system diseases.	$5–$10 a month; over the counter.

Weighing the Benefits of Human Growth Hormone Supplements

Human growth hormone (HGH) is produced by the pituitary gland at the base of the brain. It plays a vital role in bone and muscle growth as well as height.

Touted Benefits	Known Risks	Cost
Preserves lean muscle mass and skin; boosts immunity; improves heart function.	Diabetes; fluid retention; enlargement of internal organs and bones; breast enlargement in men; enlargement of head, face, hands, and feet; hypertension; and carpal tunnel syndrome. (Changes reverse when supplementation is stopped.)	$800 a month; injectable, by prescription.

Red Flag

The Dietary Supplement Health Education Act of 1994 states that the FDA (Food and Drug Administration) has no legal authority to require companies to prove that their products are effective or safe, nor does it enforce quality standards. Most supplements can be made and sold as snake oil was years ago. This means one thing—*you are not protected.* It is your right as a consumer to know that supplements are not regulated as to their claims or their potency. In other words, since supplements fall into their own category outside the regulations for food and drugs, there are *no* laws requiring that they do what they claim to do or even that the ingredients are what the label says they are!

Therefore, when buying herbal supplements, look for standardized brands. Since plants can vary significantly in their potency, the chances are greater that you will get what you pay for if you buy a brand labeled "standardized." Consult your health care provider if you are taking any prescription or over-the-counter medications as negative interactions can occur. Follow the dosage on the label carefully.

The Impotence Cure

Don't count on any of these hormones or herbs to cure impotence. The Massachusetts Male Aging Study (MMAS) looked at 1,700 Boston-area men, ages 40 to 70, and found that impotence in middle-age and older men was almost always linked to vascular conditions such as heart disease, hypertension, and diabetes. Smoking and alcoholism also increased the risk of impotence but, interestingly enough, a low testosterone level does not.

To any man, impotence is a frightening thought, yet this study revealed that more than half of all healthy men (51 percent) between the ages of 40 and 70 reported occasional to frequent problems with erection.

Step 3: Know There Is Help for Impotence

Your doctor will first try to determine whether the causes are physical, psychological, or a combination.

While researchers used to claim, "It's all in your head," today they know differently. It is now estimated that 80 percent of impotence is physical, usually resulting in reduced blood flow to the penis . . . a basic plumbing problem, if you will. Causes include the use of alcohol or drugs, ailments such as diabetes, hypertension, and heart disease, and the side effects from some medications. Did you know that one of the negative effects of antidepressants is impotence? Psychological reactions to the impotence, such as frustration and loss of self-esteem, of course, perpetuate the problem. Other reactions may include:

- Feeling down and discontent
- Anxiety and sleeplessness
- Fear
- Feelings of inadequacy

Is There Really a Cure?

Some of the most effective ways to reverse impotence include life-style changes to get healthy such as exercise, stress control, and cutting down on fat in the diet. If that is not successful, urologists have an array of options to choose from, such as the medication Viagra. This pill was scientifically designed to help men with diabetes or heart conditions, although it cannot be used in conjunction with nitroglycerin, a common medication for heart patients. There are also herbal Viagra "wannabes," many of which contain one of the following highly dangerous ingredients:

- Yohimbe: Marketed worldwide as a male aphrodisiac and cure for impotence, it can cause panic attacks and other psychological problems, as well as neurological effects that can be fatal.
- Chaparral: An American Southwestern desert bush called creosote touted for its antiaging properties but known for causing terminal liver failure.
- Ma Huang: One of several names for products containing ephedra. Common names for these evergreen plants include Mormon tea and squaw tea. Serious adverse effects include high blood pressure, nerve damage, rapid heart rate, stroke, and memory loss. Ma huang is found in both over-the-counter and prescription drugs, as well as in some weight control products.

Just the Facts

Natural doesn't always mean safe. For more information on herbs, one source to contact is the American Botanical Council at 1-800-373-7105.

Remember, you may be acting as a guinea pig for many products as we do not yet know the ultimate price that our bodies may pay. The majority of benefits at this point are usually psychological and subtle. Sometimes the only people benefiting from these hormones and herbal formulas are those who manufacture and sell them.

The Real Miracle Potion

The irony of this hormone/herbal hype is that much of what the new drug and hormones promise is readily attainable *without treatment*—and the good news is that you can start today! Exercise and a great diet can stop stress-aging by building bones and muscles, increasing strength, reducing body fat, and controlling your weight—not to mention increasing energy level and improving your mood, sleep, and libido. Exercise may even perk up production of those "stay young" hormones we so desperately seek. Your mental outlook as well as your behavior both make a huge difference in stress-aging.

Step 4: Get to Know Your Prostate

This tiny gland, which is normally about the size of a walnut, plays a key role in your physical and sexual health. Especially after age 40, your prostate can make itself known in a variety of silent but uncomfortable and even deadly ways.

BPH, or benign prostatic hyperplasia (or hypertrophy), means an enlarged prostate gland (noncancerous). When the gland is swollen, it presses against the urethra (the tube that carries urine from the bladder out the body) and makes urination painful and frequent. It may even interfere with the inability to completely empty the bladder, and as you may know, that's a very annoying feeling.

A combination of aging and changes in hormones is thought to cause BPH. Specifically, testosterone in the prostate converts into the more potent hormone DHT (dihydrotestosterone), which in large concentrations can cause cells to multiply and excessively enlarge the prostate. Medications such as Proscar and Hytrin are approved for treatment although each has negative side effects: impotence and a decreased sex drive for Proscar and dizziness and low blood pressure for Hytrin. Surgery is sometimes done to relieve the pressure on the urethra but carries the risk of leaving you incontinent or impotent.

What About Saw Palmetto?

Saw palmetto is the ripe berry of a scrubby, low-lying palm tree that grows in the southeastern United States. According to herb expert Varro Tyler, Ph.D., Sc.D., dean emeritus of the Purdue University School of Pharmacy and Pharmacal Sciences and professor emeritus of pharmacognosy, saw palmetto has been used for urinary and genital ailments for years. In European studies, saw palmetto used for three months seemed to decrease the number of nightly trips to the bathroom as well as the pain and difficulty with urination. Scientists suggest that the phytochemicals (naturally occurring plant chemicals) in saw palmetto berries help maintain a healthy prostate.

Beta-sitosterol, found naturally in soybeans, pumpkin seeds, and palmetto berries, may also help to keep your prostate healthy. This phytochemical is similar in structure to testosterone and estrogen and may block the receptor sites of these hormones and limit their effect on the prostate. Vegetarians consume more of these beneficial compounds than do meat eaters.

Just the Facts

If you decide to try saw palmetto, be sure to find a product that is standardized to provide 85 to 95 percent of the important ingredient called phytosterols. Other products, including pygeum and stinging nettle, are not as well studied for treatment of BPH as saw palmetto.

Red Flag

Never self-medicate without an exam by your health care practitioner to rule out a kidney infection, prostate cancer, or other serious illness. If you are taking saw palmetto when you go in for a PSA test (prostate-specific antigen test), tell your health care professional, as the results could be affected.

Step 5: Age-proof Your Sexual Performance and Prostate Health

Now that you know the parts of the body to pay attention to, here are ten strategies to age-proof your sexual performance:

1. Discuss taking saw palmetto with your health care professional.
2. Cut fat in your diet, especially saturated fat.
3. Eat a soy product daily, or at least 3 times a week.
4. Eat fish or shellfish for zinc and vitamin B12 a couple of times per week.
5. Include nuts and seeds (pumpkin seeds and almonds, in particular) in your diet at least 3 times a week.
6. Increase your intake of beans, peas, legumes, whole grains, and vegetables for B vitamins.

7. Take a daily vitamin-mineral supplement (choose one with a low iron level).
8. Stay flexible (your body, that is) and exercise.
9. Chill out and find time to relax.
10. Practice "safe stress"—keep that anxiety and aggression level down.

Just the Facts
Dr. John Milner and Dr. Penny Kris-Etherton, researchers at Pennsylvania State University, found that two phytochemicals in almonds known as quercetin and kaempferol were strong suppressors of lung and prostate tumor cell growth.

Not for Women Only

Now that the men know what to do to keep their engines humming, let's do some girl talk. If you are a female between the ages of 35 and 50, raise your hands if you have noticed any of the following bothersome symptoms:

Mood swings
Decrease in sexual desire
Insomnia
Night sweats
Hot flashes
Change in menstrual flow
Lowered energy level
Headaches
Vaginal dryness
Dry, itchy skin
Difficulty paying attention
Wrinkles

Now that all hands have been raised . . . let's explain that while some of these symptoms are similar to stress-aging, you could also be entering perimenopause. These are the 10 to 15 years prior to menopause, or the major decline in ovarian function. Interestingly, many women are like our friend Sara, who asked her doctor if he could predict the day menopause would happen to her because "my daughter's getting married next summer, and I don't want to have menopause on that weekend." Wow!! That's not the way this life stage works. Rather, perimenopause is a progression, not a specific date or time, not an all-or-nothing event. Unless forced by surgery or treatments such as chemotherapy, your ovaries don't just suddenly stop producing estrogen one warm day in June (although, sorry to say, you may be feeling a bit warm!). Instead, your estrogen level usually starts to decline in your late thirties, and by the mid-forties, your menstrual cycle may change (periods may become longer or shorter, heavier or lighter).

You may notice that any premenstrual symptoms become more pronounced, or they could suddenly begin, if you never had them before. Headaches are common. Hot flashes might become noticeable during the day, or you may experience night sweats that wake you up. Then, again, you may have no noticeable symptoms at all except for a decrease in menstrual flow.

"I haven't had the night sweats, but I have noticed intercourse has become painful. Could I be in menopause?" Marcy, age 41, was the mother of four children, and didn't know whether it was the results of childbirth or menopause causing this new change in her body.

Marcy's not alone. Many women report that intercourse becomes painful during the ages of 35 to 50. This could occur for a variety of reasons, including:

Hormonal changes from breast-feeding and menopause (which can be helped by our 10 top foods to tame hormones)

Eat to Stay Young

Infections such as bladder infections, yeast infections, and
STDs (sexually transmitted diseases)
Endometriosis (abnormal tissue growth in the pelvic cavity)
Nerve problems
Allergy to semen

Yet no matter how intrusive the symptoms of perimenopause
or menopause may be, there is a better way. We know that you
can gain control over many of these feelings using the EAT Plan.
No, we don't mean that every time you have a hot flash you are
to douse the flames with an ice cream sundae! Rather, there are
some scientifically proven foods you can enjoy in this life stage
that will help soothe hormone havoc.

Step 1: EAT to Calm the Storm

While the argument continues over the pros and cons of hormone
replacement therapy (discussed on page 247) look to your diet for
help. Diet is a first-line approach to perimenopause and menopause.
Phytoestrogens are naturally occurring compounds in plants that
mimic the effect of estrogen in the body and can play an important
role in the management of menopausal complaints. The most common phytoestrogens are isoflavones, flavones, and lignins.

The Lowdown on Soy

Vegetarians have known for years that soy protein is an easy,
inexpensive, and healthy alternative to meat. Soy products are
lactose free, cholesterol free, packed with phytoestrogens, and
are low in saturated fat. For years, soybeans have played an
integral part in the Asian diet. In fact, heart disease, breast cancer,
prostate cancer, and osteoporosis rates for Asian men and women
are much lower than for Americans. In a recent study of 1,000

people reported in the *American Journal of Epidemiology* (1996), those who ate soybeans in some form at least once a week had half the risk of developing the polyps that are precursors to colon cancer compared to those who did not eat soybeans. In addition, the isoflavones in soy appear to have no harmful side effects and can help relieve the menopausal symptoms that frequently occur because of plummeting estrogen levels.

Studies show that soy can also effectively help prevent the rise in serum cholesterol associated with a declining estrogen level as well as possibly reduce the risk of certain cancers and osteoporosis. Many studies are in progress to determine whether it is the soy protein, the isoflavones, or a combination of both that provide these potentially wonderful benefits.

Anatomy 101

Isoflavones are phytochemicals found in soy that act as phytoestrogens (plant estrogens that are close in structure to the body's form of estrogen) in the body.

The Latest in Soy Products

When you think of soy, do you think of a blob of white stuff that has no flavor? If all you know about soy is limited to tofu and you aren't so keen on tofu (or maybe you're not quite sure what to do with it), prepare to be pleasantly surprised. Over the past decade more than 2,000 new soy products were introduced to consumers, including meatless pepperoni, salami, hot dogs, and bacon as well as puddings and dairy alternatives. You can also find calcium-rich soy foods such as tahini, calcium-set tofu, fortified soy milk, textured vegetable protein, and soy nuts.

The following soy products represent just a few that are available at supermarkets, natural food stores, and Asian markets:

Soy Superstars

Food	Serving	Isoflavones (mg)*
Roasted soy nuts	¼ cup	62
Tempeh	½ cup	35
Low-fat tofu	½ cup	35
Regular tofu	½ cup	35
Soy milk	1 cup	30
Low-fat soy milk	1 cup	20

*Aim for 30 to 60 mg per day.

Isolated Soy Protein: This is a powder form of soy protein that you can add to casseroles, pasta dishes, smoothie drinks, and more. One ounce contains approximately 23 grams of soy protein and has little effect on taste.

Miso: This rich, salty paste made from soybeans and grains is aged for 1 to 3 years in wooden vats. Used to flavor soups, sauces, and marinades, miso can taste delicate and sweet or savory and salty. While miso contains isoflavones, since the typical serving size is small (1 teaspoon), you only get a minimal benefit.

Soybeans: These dried soybeans have a delicious nutty flavor and can be used in recipes such as baked beans or chili. Just remember to soak them first as you would any dried bean. You can add to soups or use in any recipe that calls for lentils. One-half cup provides 14.3 grams of soy protein.

Soy flour: Made from roasted soybeans that are ground into a very fine powder, soy flour can be purchased in defatted, low-fat, or full-fat versions. One-half cup of full-fat soy flour contains 15 grams of soy protein, while the defatted soy flour has 24 grams of soy protein. Use soy flour to replace up to one-fourth of regular flour in recipes.

Soy granules: These are tasty, nutty granules that shake directly out of the container. You can soak these, then use as a filler in recipes or sprinkle directly on food such as ice cream or yogurt. Soy granules have 23 grams of soy protein per one-fourth cup.

Soy milk: This liquid can be used in virtually any recipe that calls for milk, and the added benefit is that 8 ounces contain approximately 10 grams of soy protein. Be sure and look for soy milk that is calcium-fortified.

Tempeh: This thin cake is made from fermented soybeans. It has an interesting nutty or smokey taste and a chewy texture; 4 ounces contain almost 17 grams of soy protein. Tempeh is frequently used as a substitute for beef and contains more whole soybeans and fiber than soy milk or tofu.

Textured soy protein (TSP): This is a quick-cooking meat substitute made from low-fat soy flour that can be used for burgers, chili, sloppy joes, and more. It is available in many forms including strips, chunks, flakes, and granules. One half-cup serving has 11 grams of soy protein. Note, however, that some processed soy foods such as this have had the isoflavones removed.

Tofu: This soy product is also called bean curd. It is a tasteless food, but by blending it with herbs, spices, and other foods, it becomes very appetizing. Tofu comes in a myriad of varieties, including soft, firm, extra firm, and silken, and is available in regular and low-fat forms, too. You can use tofu to replace a portion or all sour cream or cream cheese, mix it in stir fry, smoothies, puddings or a mousse. Four ounces of firm tofu contains 9 to 13 grams of soy protein; the same amount of soft tofu contains 9 grams of soy protein. Watch out for the fat in tofu. A 3-ounce portion of ''lite'' tofu contains about 1 gram of fat while the same portion of regular firm tofu contains up to 7 grams.

Just the Facts

For more information on soy, go to website:http://www.soy-foods.com or call the Soyfoods Center at 510-283-2991.

Lingo Lowdown

Bioflavonoids are another group of estrogen compounds found in citrus fruits, grape skins, cherry skins, and in supplement form.

EFAs (essential fatty acids) such as linolenic acid help keep skin, vaginal tissue, and other mucous membranes healthy. Linolenic acid (an omega-3 fatty acid) can be found in fish, flaxseed, pumpkin seeds, and walnuts.

Top Ten Foods to Tame Raging Hormones

Based on what you have just read, we have compiled our list of the top ten foods both sexes can eat to calm hormone havoc.

1. Flaxseed (2–3 tablespoons per day—look for it in breads or ground as meal for sprinkling on cereal, yogurt, or in cooking)
2. Walnuts
3. Pumpkin seeds
4. Fish and shellfish
5. Grapes
6. Cherries
7. Citrus fruits

8. Soy foods
9. Sweet potatoes
10. Calcium-rich foods (dairy foods, calcium-fortified products, and vegetables)

Just the Facts
According to Robert Heaney, M.D., professor of medicine at Creighton University, adding skim milk to your coffee can offset the loss of calcium from the body caused by caffeine. Better yet, order a cappuccino made with skim milk and be even farther ahead of the game.

Speaking of calcium, men and women can bone up with these calcium-containing vegetables:

Butternut squash	Snap beans
Broccoli	Lima beans
Cabbage	Carrots
Artichokes	Spinach
Brussels sprouts	Swiss chard

Step 2: Weigh the Benefits and Risks of Hormone Replacement Therapy

If you haven't already done so, ask your doctor for a complete physical to determine if perimenopause or menopause is the cause of your symptoms. If the cause is hormonal, hormone replacement therapy (HRT) may be recommended. However, only about 30 percent of perimenopausal and postmenopausal women use HRT and fewer than one third of them are on it at the end of three years due to side effects. Note, however, that most of the time, these annoying side effects, such as heavier menstrual cycles, weight gain, or break-through bleeding, can be corrected by using a different brand, different form, or lower dose, or by altering the usage schedule.

Fewer than half the women who could benefit from hormone replacement therapy are taking it, due in part to concerns over breast cancer, and are looking instead to alternative therapies. The National Institute of Aging is taking a broad look at the influence of diet on women's health through its multicenter Study of Women's Health Across the Nation (SWAN). Researchers are also evaluating various supplements, teas, and herbs, particularly looking at the estrogenic effects by measuring blood levels of estrogens and phytoestrogens. Rigorous, large-scale studies are needed to determine safe levels and combinations of herbal remedies that are beneficial.

Weigh the Benefits of HRT

- Helps prevent wrinkles. HRT is great for the skin, and many women notice stronger nails and thicker hair as well. However, sometimes side effects such as melasma (patches of darker, irregular skin pigmentation) and acne can also be a problem. If this is a concern ask your health care provider to change the dosage or type of hormones. Or try bleaching creams or other products to reduce the skin problems.
- Reduces symptoms of menopause such as hot flashes and vaginal drying.
- Protects bone health (even teeth).
- Preserves blood vessel flexibility, helping to prevent heart disease.
- May help prevent Alzheimer's disease. Scientists from the Baltimore Longitudinal Study of Aging found a 54 percent reduction in Alzheimer's risk in women who had taken estrogen.
- Lowers LDL cholesterol and boosts HDL cholesterol.

- May offer protection against colon cancer and rheumatoid arthritis.
- Could reduce the progression of Parkinson's disease.
- Reduces dry mouth and gingivitis associated with menopause.
- May aid in wound healing. Researchers from the University of Florida found that postmenopausal women taking HRT had wounds that healed at much the same rate as younger women while the postmenopausal patients not taking HRT showed delayed wound healing. There was also more collagen at the wound site in women on HRT.

Weigh the Risks

- May increase breast cancer risk.
- Could bring back your period, depending on whether estrogen and progesterone are taken together.
- May increase risk of asthma.

Step 3: Discuss the Use of Testosterone with Your Physician

"What about testosterone for women? Wouldn't this help with a low sex drive?" Yes, definitely. Some women who take HRT may experience symptoms such as a low energy level and a sex drive stuck in neutral. Some researchers now suggest that a small amount of testosterone added to their HRT may be just the magic potion! Women's ovaries and adrenal glands do provide a modest amount of testosterone but that amount is severely lowered after menopause. If you decide to take testosterone, watch out for the side effects, ranging from acne and oily skin to hair growth on the body, high blood pressure, and an increase in heart disease risk.

Step 4: Try Herbal Therapies

Whether for medical or personal reasons, many women choose not to use HRT and seek out herbal remedies. There are a number of products on the market that are considered both safe and effective, along with a bunch that are merely a sham. Although many studies are currently underway in the United States to evaluate the safety and effectiveness of herbs for menopause, some herbs have been safely used in Germany for many years. The German Commission E is Germany's leading authority in the evaluation of herbal remedies for safety and effectiveness and much of our information comes from them. Note: While the effectiveness of certain herbs for menopausal symptoms has been confirmed, we don't know yet whether these natural products offer the same health benefits as HRT, such as protection against heart disease, osteoporosis, Alzheimer's disease or Parkinson's disease.

Just the Facts

German Commission E is Germany's leading authority in the evaluation of herbal remedies for safety and effectiveness. For a leading reference in the United States, check out *The Honest Herbal* by Varro Tyler, Ph.D., Sc.D., dean emeritus of the Purdue University School of Pharmacy.

Herbs for Hormone Havoc

If you prefer the natural cure, here are some herbs that may be worth a try to ease your symptoms:

- Black cohosh: Possibly relieves night sweats and hot flashes, headaches, vaginal drying, and heart palpitations. The herb suppresses the secretion of luteinizing hormone

(LH), thought to be involved in many of these symptoms. Approved for treatment of menopausal symptoms by German Commission E. Available in capsules, tablets, and drops. One brand, Remifemin, has been around for decades in Europe and is now in the United States. Long-term toxicity has not been evaluated so experts suggest you use it for only 6 months at a time, with breaks in between. Forty milligrams per day is the usual dosage.

* Valerian: Easily brewed as tea and may be helpful for irritability and restlessness by working as a mild tranquilizer and sleep aid.

* Red clover: A plant that contains the phytoestrogens isoflavones and flavones, which can ease the symptoms of menopause. It is touted to have a higher isoflavone level than soy. Suggested dosage is 500 milligrams a day with a meal.

Don't Add Fuel to Your Fire

The following are popular remedies that need a word of caution. After all, sometimes the symptoms of menopause are disturbing enough without having to deal with unwanted or even dangerous side effects of herbal treatments.

* Dong quai or dong kway: Although very popular in Chinese traditional medicine, it has not been evaluated by Western methods. At this point, no phytoestrogenic effect has been documented. According to Dr. Varro Tyler, the volatile oil in the herb can relax the uterus, but a water extract form of the plant does just the opposite—it stimulates the uterus. Take caution with sun exposure as this herb makes you more sun sensitive.

* Chasteberry: Touted to relieve hot flashes, headaches, heart

palpitations, and vaginal drying. Dosage recommendation is 20 milligrams per day and can be made as a tea. Although approved by Commission E, Dr. Tyler suspects that the herb's chemical composition is more suited for PMS symptoms.

Chasteberry is not for use by women who are experiencing a lowered sex drive, as the herbal literature suggests it is likely to reduce sexual desire.

- Ginseng: Touted as an antiaging herb that improves sexual performance, tones your skin, and prevents fine lines (if applied topically). Ginseng might smooth away some of the slight depression and fatigue associated with menopause. It is a stimulant that may boost feelings of well-being but evidence for relief of specific symptoms is mainly anecdotal at this point. Note: A survey of over 50 ginseng products found that 60 percent contained such small amounts of ginseng that they were considered inactive. The majority of studies to date have been done on *Panax* (scientific name or genus) ginseng and would be the best bet if you choose to try it.

Red Flag

Some herbal extracts may contain up to 55 percent alcohol, so read the label carefully.

Step 5: Consider SERMs Instead of HRT

The next generation of HRT are compounds known as SERMs (selective estrogen-receptor modulators). It was previously thought that if you took estrogen, it would affect all of your body—breasts, bones, hips—the same way. However, when the estrogen drug tamoxifen was being tested, it was found that the estrogen was going not to the breast but to the bone. What does this mean to you? It means that perhaps estrogen doesn't work the same way in every cell and maybe compounds can be developed that are tissue specific. Another drug, raloxifene, may offer many of estrogen's benefits, such as protecting your heart and bones, without the risk of breast or uterine cancer.

Step 6: Pump Up Your Sex Life

The easiest way to enjoy sex—no matter what your age—is *not* found in an herb or prescription. It's in the Kegel. This is an exercise that not only tones your vaginal muscles but may help lubricate the vagina, and it's easy to learn. While you are sitting on the toilet, stop the flow of urine. Then relax and let the urine stream continue. These are the muscles you want to strengthen. Lying down, sitting, or standing, contract and relax, hold each contraction for 10 seconds. If you could easily stop and start the flow, then 20 to 25 contractions per day should keep you in good sexual form. If you had a hard time stopping the flow of urine, do 50 contractions a day (divided into 2 or 3 sessions).

Lastly, if your sex life is in the dump, it's time to get off the roller coaster of life and make time to revitalize and get some exercise. After all, the EAT Plan is all about making time for ourselves and what better way than pausing to do something healthful like exercise? A pilot study at the University of Michigan Division of Kinesiology suggests that higher-intensity exercise in postmenopausal women may cause them to secrete more growth hormone. Remember, growth hormone helps with bone formation and reduces the effects of aging. This was a small study but certainly warrants further investigation on a larger scale! It is also suspected that you can increase your HGH level with both weight lifting and running (see Age Deactivator 4).

Finale

B.R.A.V.O. for You!

As you take advantage of the host of stress-aging information in this book and follow the six-step EAT Plan, you are well on your way to staying young. We have demonstrated that no matter how stressed you are, you can stop stress-aging.

Yet when you feel as if you cannot muster the strength to follow the EAT Plan, we want you to consider the following:

Belief: Believe that you can start over and reach your goals to feel young again.

Responsibility: No one can take responsibility for deactivating stress-aging but you.

Action: Don't forget that commitment can follow behavior. Launch out toward your goals, and usually your ''feelings'' will follow.

Vision: Practice the visualization techniques described on page 216, and imagine how wonderful you are going to look and feel when you get fully immersed in the EAT Plan for the rest of your life.

Opportunity: See the EAT Plan as an opportunity of a lifetime!

B.R.A.V.O.!

If you can do these steps, then we applaud you, saying "B.R.A.V.O.!" This method of determining goals and learning ways to keep them (without punishing yourself when you slip) will enable you to enjoy your small successes along the way and feel a sense of accomplishment as you reach each new goal.

It's all up to you. Perhaps Henry Ford said it best: "Whether you believe you can or believe you can't, you're right!"

References and Supporting Research

Age differences in stress, coping, and appraisal: findings from the normative aging study. *The Journal of Gerontology,* Series B, July 1996; 51(4): P179(10).

Ainlay, S.C. et al. Aging and religious participation: reconsidering the effects of health. *Journal for the Scientific Study of Religion,* 1992; 31: 175–188.

Alpert, J.E. et al. Nutrition and depression: the role of folate. *Nutrition Reviews,* 1997; 55(5): 145–149.

American Dietetic Association 1997 Nutrition Trends Survey, American Dietetic Association, September 1997.

Ancoli-Israel, S. Sleep problems in older adults: putting myths to bed. *Geriatrics,* 1997; 52(19): 20–30.

Bartels, C.L. and Miller, S.J. Herbal and related remedies. *Nutrition in Clinical Practice,* 1998; 12(2): 5–19.

Beisel, W. History of nutritional immunology: introduction and overview. *Journal of Nutrition,* 1992; 122: 591–596.

Benson, H. and Stark, M. "Reason to Believe." *Natural Health,* May—June 1996, 74.

Bienenfeld, M.D. et al. Psychosocial predictors of mental health in a population of elderly women: test of an explanatory model. *American Journal of Geriatric Psychiatry,* 1997; 5: 43–53.

Bjorntorp, P. Neuroendocrine aging. *Journal of Internal Medicine,* 1995; 238(5): 401–4.

Borysenko, J. *Minding the Body, Mending the Mind* (Reading, MA: Addison-Wesley, 1987), 10.

Burns-Cox, N. and Gingell C. The andropause: fact or fiction? *Postgraduate Medical Journal,* 1997; 73(863): 553–56.

Callahan, M. Antioxidants and fewer health problems. *Bottom Line Personal,* Jan. 15, 1996, 8.

Camara, E.G. and Danao, T.C. The brain and the immune system. *Psychosomatics,* 1989; 30(2): 140–48.

Chandra, R.K. Nutrition and the immune system: an introduction. *American Journal of Clinical Nutrition,* 1997; 66(2): 460S–63S.

Chew, B.P. Antioxidant vitamins affect food animal immunity and health. *Journal of Nutrition,* June 1995; 125(6 Suppl): 1804s–8s.

Clamlan, H.N. The biology of the immune response. *Journal of the American Medical Association,* 1992; 268(20): 2790–801.

Cohen, S. et al. Psychological stress and susceptibility to the common cold. *New England Journal of Medicine,* 1991; 325: 606–12.

Cohen, S. et al. Social ties and susceptibility to the common cold. *New England Journal of Medicine,* 1997; 277(24): 1940–44.

Cohen, S. and Herbert T.B. (1996). Health psychology: psychological factors and physical disease from the perspective of human psychoneuroimmunology. *Annual Reviews in Psychology,* 1996; 47: 113–42.

Coping with stress: a physician's guide to mental health in aging. *Geriatrics,* July 1996; 51(7): 46(4).

Cortisol, ACTH, and cardiovascular response to a cognitive challenge paradigm in aging and depression. *The American Journal of Physiology,* April 1995; 268(4): R865(9).

Dementia, aging, and the stress control system (Commentary). *The Lancet,* March 18, 1995; 345 (8951): 666(2).

Does age affect the stress and coping process? Implications of age differences in perceived control. *Journal of Gerontology,* July 1991; 46(4): P174(7).

Dorsey, C.M. et al. Effects of passive body heating on the sleep of older female insomniacs. *Journal of Geriatric Psychiatry and Neurology,* 1996; 9(2): 83–90.

Dossey, L. *Healing Words.* HarperCollins, 1993, 38.

Drewnowski, A. et al. Taste responses to naringin, a flavonoid, and the acceptance of grapefruit juice are related to genetic sensitivity to 6-n-propylthiouraci. *American Journal of Clinical Nutrition,* 1997; 66: 391–97.

Esterling, B.A. et al. Psychosocial modulation of cytokine-induced natural killer cell activity in older adults. *Psychosomatic Medicine,* 1996; 58(3): 264–72.

Evans, W.J. Exercise, nutrition, and aging. *Clinical Geriatric Medicine,* 1995; 11(4): 725–34.

Foltz-Gray, D. My happiness gene. *Health.* Sept. 1997; 60–62.

Gallup Institute. Religion in America—50 years. (Princeton, NJ: Princeton Religious Research Center, 1995).

Goodman, M. et al. Hostility predicts rustiness after percutaneous transluminal coronary angioplasty. *Mayo Clinic Proceedings,* 1996; 71: 729–34.

Gordon N. Life style exercise: a new strategy to promote physical activity for adults. *Journal of Cardiopulmonary Rehabilitation,* 1993; 13: 161–63.

Grodstein, F. et al. Three-year follow-up of participants in a commercial weight loss program. Can you keep it off? *Archives of Internal Medicine,* 1996; 156(12): 1302–6.

Gupta V. and Korte, C. The effect of a confidant and a peer group on the well-being of senior elders. *International Journal of Aging and Human Development,* 1994; 39(4): 293–302.

Hafen, B.O. et al. *Health Effects of Attitudes, Emotions and Relationships.* (Utah: EMS Associates, 1992).

Hall, M. et al. Disruption in sleep decreases natural killer cells. *Psychosomatic Medicine,* Jan. 23, 1998.

Hall, N., ed. *Mind Body Interactions and Disease and Psychoneuroimmunological Aspects of Health and Disease.* (Orlando: Health Dateline Press, 1996).

Healthscan: Advice to power walkers. *Cooking Light,* March 1996; 17.

Hirsch, C. "Insidious allergies caused by immune system's overreaction." *Health News and Review,* Winter 1995; 9(2).

Hoffman-Goetz, L. Influence of physical activity and exercise on innate immunity. *Nutrition Reviews,* 1998; 56(1): S126–30.

House, J.S. et al. Social relationships and health. *Science,* 1988; 241: 540.

Jaret, P. You don't have to sweat to reduce your stress. *Health,* November/December 1995; 83–88.

Jorgenson, J. Therapeutic use of companion animals in health care. *Image J Nurs Sch,* 1997; 29(3): 249–54.

Keefe, F.J. et al. Pain in arthritis and musculoskeletal disorders: the role of coping skills training and exercise interventions. *Journal of Orthopedic Sports and Physical Therapy,* 1996; 24(4): 279–90.

Kendler, K.S. Religion, psychopathology, and substance use and abuse: a multimeasure, genetic-epidemiologic study. *American Journal of Psychiatry,* 1997; 154: 322–29.

Kendler, K.S. Social support: a genetic-epidemiologic analysis. *American Journal of Psychiatry,* Oct. 1997; 154: 1398–1404.

Key, T.J.A. et al. *British Medical Journal,* 1996; 313: 1–13.

Kiecolt-Glaser, J.K. et al. Marital conflict and endocrine function: are men really more physiologically affected than women? *Journal of Consulting and Clinical Psychology,* 1996; 64(2): 324–32.

Kiecolt-Glaser, J.K. et al. Chronic stress alters the immune response to influenza virus vaccine in older adults. *Proceedings of the National Academy of Science, USA,* 1996; 93(7): 3043–47.

Koenig, H.G. et al. Modeling the cross-sectional relationships between religion, physical health, social support, and depressive symptoms. *American Journal of Geriatric Psychiatry,* 1997; 5: 131–44.

Kraemer, W.J. and Koziris, L.P. Muscle strength training: techniques and considerations. *Physical Therapy Practice,* 1992; 2(1): 54–68.

Krause, K.R. and Van Tran, T. Stress and religious involvement among older blacks. *Journal of Gerontology,* 1989; 44: S4–13.

Kujala, U.M. et al. Relationship of leisure-time physical activity and mortality. *Journal of the American Medical Association,* 1998; 279(6): 440–44.

Lachance, P. *Journal of the American College of Nutrition,* October 1997.

Landeman, L.R. et al. Alternative models of the stress-buffering hypothesis. *American Journal of Community Psychology,* 1989; 17: 625–42.

Lane, M.A. et al. Dehydroepiandrosyerone sulfate: a biomarker of primate aging slowed by calorie restriction. *Journal of Clinical Endocrinology and Metabolism,* July 1997; 82(7): 2093–96.

Le Bars, P.L. et al. A placebo-controlled, double-blind, randomized trial of an extract of Ginkgo biloba for dementia. *Journal of the American Medical Association,* 1997; 278: 1327–32.

Levin, J.S. Religion and health: is there an association, is it valid, and is it causal? *Social Science Medicine,* 1994; 38: 1475–82.

Luecken, L.J. et al. Stress in employed women: impact of marital status and children at home on neurohormone output and home strain. *Psychosomatic Medicine,* 1997; 59(4): 352–59.

Maton, K.I. The stress buffering role of spiritual support: cross-sectional and prospective investigation. *Journal of Scientific Study of Religion,* 1989; 28: 310–23.

McGrady, A. et al. The effects of biofeedback-assisted relaxation on cell-mediated immunity, cortisol, and white blood cell count in healthy adult subjects. *Journal of Behavioral Medicine,* 1992; 15(4): 343–54.

Mead, N. Mind/body answer to allergies. *Natural Health,* September–October 1995; 25(5): 58(4).

Miller, C. Mental powers: divine power over blood pressure. *Longevity,* September 1989, 78.

Modica. P. The ancient art of acupuncture gets FDA approval. *Medical Tribune News Service,* May 24, 1996.

Moore, T. *Care of the Soul: A Guide for Cultivating Depth and Sacredness in Everyday Life* (HarperCollins, 1992).

Morris, J.F. Physiologic Changes Due to Age. *Drugs and Aging,* 1994; 4: 207–20.

Moss, R.B. et al. Microstress, mood and natural killer-cell activity. *Psychosomatics,* 1989; 30(3): 279–83.

Nehlsen-Cannarella S.L. et al. The effects of moderate exercise training on immune response. *Medicine and Science in Sports and Exercise,* 1991; 23(1): 64–70.

Newton, T.L. and Kiecolt-Glaser, J.K. Hostility and erosion of marital quality during early marriage. *Journal of Behavioral Medicine,* 1995; 18(6): 601–19.

Nielsen, H.B. et al. Lymphocytes and NK cell activity during repeated bouts of maximal exercise. *American Journal of Physiology,* 1996; 40: R222–27.

Nieman, D.C. et al. Moderate exercise training and natural killer cell cytotoxic activity in breast cancer patients. *International Journal of Sports Medicine,* 1995b; 16: 334–47.

Osiewacz, H.D. Genetic regulation of aging. *Journal of Molecular Medicine,* 1997; 75(10): 715–27.

Pedersen, B.K. and Brunnsgaard, H. How physical exercise influences the establishment of infections. *Sports Medicine,* 1995; 19: 393–400.

Pollack, M.L. et al. Effect of age and training on aerobic capacity and body composition of master athletes. *Journal of Applied Physiology,* 1987; 62: 725–31.

Rainey, C. et al. The California avocado. *Nutrition Today,* 1994; 29(3): 23–27.

Reilly, D. et al. Is evidence for homeopathy reproducible? *Lancet,* December 10, 1994; 344 (8937): 1601(6).

Sabate, J. et al. Effects of walnuts on serum lipid levels and blood pressure in normal men. *New England Journal of Medicine,* 1993; 328: 603–7.

Salivary cortisol levels and stress reactivity in human aging. *The Journal of Gerontology,* Series A, March 1997; 52(2): M68(8).

Sato, Y. et al. Effects of long-term psychological stress on sexual behavior and brain catecholamine levels. *Journal of Andrology,* 1996; 17(2): 83–90.

Schulz, P. et al. Lower sex hormones in men during anticipatory stress. *Neuroreport,* 1996; 7(18): 3101–4.

Siegler, H.C. et al. Personality factors differentially predict exercise behavior in men and women. *Women's Health,* 1997; 3(1): 61–70.

Singh, N.A. et al. A randomized controlled trial of the effect of exercise on sleep. *Sleep,* 1997; 20(2): 95–101.

Skolnick, A.A. Scientific verdict still out on DHEA. *Journal of the American Medical Association,* 1996; 276(17): 1365–67.

Stress and neuroendocrine changes during aging. *Generations,* Fall-Winter 1992; 16(4): 35(4).

Thomson, K.S. The revival of experiments on prayer. *American Scientist,* 1996; 84: 532–34.

The influence of age on endocrine responses to ultraendurance stress. *Journal of Gerontology,* July 1993; 48(4): M134(6).

Tyler, V.E. *Herbs of Choice: The Therapeutic Use of Phytomedicinals.* (New York: Pharmaceutical Products Press [Haworth Press], 1994).

Tyler, V.E. *The Honest Herbal: A Sensible Guide to the Use of Herbs and Related Remedies.* Third Edition. (New York: Pharmaceutical Products Press, [Haworth Press], 1993).

Uchino, B.N. et al. The relationship between social support and physiological processes: a review with emphasis on underlying mechanisms and implications for health. *Psychological Bulletin,* 1996; 119(3): 488–531.

Valdimarsdottir, H.B. and Stone, A.A. Psychosocial factors and secretory immunoglobulin A. *Critical Reviews of Biological Medicine,* 1997; 8(4): 461–74.

Wang, H. et al. Total antioxidant capacity of fruits. *Journal of Agricultural and Food Chemistry,* 1996; 44(3): 701–5.

Wright, K.P. et al. Caffeine and light effects on nighttime melatonin and temperature levels in sleep-deprived humans. *Brain Research,* 1997; 747(19): 78–84.

Your skin: stress & fitness. *Total Health,* October 1995; 17(5): 46(3).

Supplemental Resources

American Herbal Pharmacopoeia (AHP), R. Upton, editor
Box 5159
Santa Cruz, CA 95063
408-461-6317

Handbook of Medicinal Herbs, J.A. Duke
CRC Press, 1985
Boca Raton, FL

German Commission E Monographs, M. Blumenthal et al. editors
American Botanical Council
PO Box 201660
Austin, TX 78720
512-331-8868

HerbalGram Journal of the American Botanical Council and the Herb Research Foundation, M. Blumenthal, editor
    American Botanical Council
    PO Box 201660
    Austin, TX 78720
    512-331-8868

Herbal Medicines: A Guide for the Health Care Professional, C. Newall, Anderson, and J. Phillipson
    The Pharmaceutical Press, 1996
    London

Herbs of Choice: The Therapeutic Use of Phytomedicines, V.E. Tyler
    Pharmaceutical Products Press (Haworth Press), 1994
    Binghampton, NY

Herbal Drugs and Phytopharmaceuticals, N.G. Bisset, editor
    CRC Press, 1994
    Boca Raton, FL

The Honest Herbal, 3rd edition, V.E. Tyler
    Pharmaceutical Products Press (Haworth Press), 1993
    Binghampton, NY

Lawrence Review of Natural Products, B.R. Loin, editor
    Facts and Comparisons, 1997
    St. Louis, MO

Rational Phytotherapy, V. Schultz, R. Hansel, and V.E. Tyler
    Springer, 1997
    Berlin

Index